Understanding Menopause

was written to help women deal with the apprehension and fear that many face as they approach menopause by offering them clear, useful information and genuine support and caring. In addition to up-to-date medical information, this book addresses a woman's psychological and emotional state during menopause, providing information on midlife relationships and the aging process.

Understanding Menopause

is the definitive guide for every woman about to experience the "change of life." Its clear nonmedical language and comforting tone will help women to realize that menopause can be a time of personal growth and positive change.

Janine O'Leary Cobb is the fou.... and editor of *A Friend Indeed*, a monthly newsletter for women in the prime of life. An internationally recognized expert on menopause, she has appeared on dozens of radio and television shows and testified on the subject of health care for women at midlife for the Congressional Subcommittee on Housing and Consumer Interests. Now often called "The Menopause Lady," she is a former professor of humanities and sociology at Vanier College. She lives in Montreal, Canada.

Understanding Menopause

Answers and Advice for Women in the Prime of Life

Janine O'Leary Cobb

A PLUME BOOK

PUBLISHER'S NOTE

The ideas, procedures, and suggestions contained in this book are not intended as a substitute for consulting with your physician. All matters regarding your health require medical supervision.

PLUME
Published by the Penguin Group
Penguin Books USA Inc., 375 Hudson Street, New York, New York 10014, U.S.A.
Penguin Books Ltd, 27 Wrights Lane, London W8 5TZ, England
Penguin Books Australia Ltd, Ringwood, Victoria, Australia
Penguin Books Canada Ltd, 10 Alcorn Avenue, Toronto, Ontario, Canada M4V 3B2
Penguin Books (N.Z.) Ltd, 182-190 Wairau Road, Auckland 10, New Zealand

Penguin Books Ltd, Registered Offices: Harmondsworth, Middlesex, England

First published in the United States of America by Plume, an imprint of Dutton Signet, a division of Penguin Books USA Inc. Originally published in a different form in Canada by Key Porter Books.

First Plume Printing, September, 1993
10 9 8 7 6 5 4 3

Copyright © Key Porter Books, 1988
Copyright © Janine O'Leary Cobb, 1993
All rights reserved.

 REGISTERED TRADEMARK—MARCA REGISTRADA

LIBRARY OF CONGRESS CATALOGING IN PUBLICATION DATA
Cobb, Janine O'Leary.
  Understanding Menopause / Janine O'Leary Cobb.
    p. cm.
  Includes bibliographical references and index.
  ISBN 0-452-27028-6
  1. Menopause—Popular works. I. Title.
RG186.C62 1993
612.6'63—dc20   93-12308
                                                       CIP

Printed in the United States of America
Set in Century Expanded
Designed by Eve L. Kirch

Without limiting the rights under copyright reserved above, no part of this publication may be reproduced, stored in or introduced into a retrieval system, or transmitted, in any form, or by any means (electronic, mechanical, photocopying, recording, or otherwise), without the prior written permission of both the copyright owner and the above publisher of this book.

BOOKS ARE AVAILABLE AT QUANTITY DISCOUNTS WHEN USED TO PROMOTE PRODUCTS OR SERVICES. FOR INFORMATION PLEASE WRITE TO PREMIUM MARKETING DIVISION, PENGUIN BOOKS USA INC., 375 HUDSON STREET, NEW YORK, NEW YORK 10014.

Contents

Introduction

It was my intention that my forty-ninth summer be memorable. I planned to spend most of that summer in the country, taking possession of the cottage that we had planned and dreamed about for years. I also intended to give up smoking—this time for good—as a fiftieth birthday present to myself, and to write a text for a course I had been developing for my classes at Vanier College in Montreal. I had been smoking steadily and heavily for almost thirty years; I needed a peaceful and ordered existence if I were to stop smoking and write a book. Fortunately, four of the five children had summer jobs or were away at camp; the youngest would be pleasant company during the week and my husband would arrive on Friday afternoons for the weekend.

The cottage got built, the manuscript was finished, and I haven't smoked since, but that summer is memorable for other reasons. I remember the sudden fits of warmth during the night (except for pregnancy, I had never been *too* warm!), the aching right shoulder (which forced me to swim sidestroke when I preferred the Australian crawl), and the weird dreams of giving birth or of waking to a bed flooded with menstrual fluid. I didn't realize it at the time, but the summer constituted a turning point—an unconscious farewell to the closure of my reproductive life.

Over the following academic year, I continued to teach. The usual routine of preparation, classes, and marking was overshadowed by threatened changes to the college system—changes that would drastically increase the numbers of students in the classroom and, at the same time, shrink the amount of time available for classroom preparation and grading. I was also coping with a full house: the two eldest, who had been away from home working or traveling, returned to go back to school. I thought I would never live through Christmas with all its attendant responsibilities. By the time classes got underway in January, I was in the throes of a full-fledged depression.

Because I was still menstruating, I never seriously thought of menopause. I believed (from what little I knew) that menopause was a problem only to women who had time on their hands. As a full-time college professor, wife, and mother, I had no time for menopausal distress. When I complained about my lagging capacity for coping, I discovered that most of my same-age friends were feeling much the same. Some were having serious problems with children; some were making noises about leaving their husbands; all were talking about burnout and the inability to feel enthusiastic about their jobs. And *none* of us attributed any of this to menopause.

In June 1983, I celebrated my fiftieth birthday in the South of France—my first trip to Europe and a glorious birthday present from a husband who was, by this time, turning cartwheels in an effort to cheer me up. I continued to feel grim—weepy and pessimistic about everything—but I wouldn't see a doctor because I was convinced I had no *reason* to feel depressed. I refused to discuss the matter, and I grew accustomed to the strange glances from family members.

By Christmas of that year (the year we bought a computer as a gift for the children), I had done a bit of research

on menopause. I had browsed through the Health section
of the bookstores. looking for a paragraph, a chapter—
something that would give me a clue. I had found some interesting material (e.g., Rosetta Reitz's book, *Menopause: A
Positive Approach,* and a chapter in Penny Wise Budoff's
first book, *No More Menstrual Cramps and Other Good
News),* but I was beginning to get angry about the general
lack of information. At my annual checkup, the doctor had
mentioned a discussion group on menopause, adding that it
was primarily informational (information that I had already
found for myself), but that it might provide moral support. I
didn't have time to register or to attend—I was about to
start a course in word processing. As I became familiar with
the capabilities of the computer, it all started to come together.

I got the idea for a newsletter for menopausal women,
which could be both a source of information and a support
group *through the mail* for women, like me, who had no time
in their lives to organize or attend a support group. In March
1984, I carefully printed out a prototype newsletter, mailing
it to any and every woman I had ever met or heard about
who might be interested. Because menopause was a time
when a woman often *is* in need, I called it *A Friend Indeed.*

Since that first tentative mailing to forty women, *A
Friend Indeed* has grown steadily. During that summer, a
newspaper article about the newsletter was reprinted across
the country; a week later, I received more than 900 enquir-
ies. (The mailman appeared on my front porch one day with
two large sacks of mail in his hands and a quizzical look on
his face: "Just what have you been *doing,* Mrs. Cobb?") The
personal stories contained in those letters were enough to
convince me that this is where I was most needed.

In October 1984, I attended my first International Congress on the Menopause where I learned how gynecologists
regarded menopause and where I met other women active
in menopause research, many of whom have since become
good friends. We are all part of a growing network of women

who are fighting to have menopause recognized—*not* as a syndrome, or deficiency, or disease, but as a natural stage of life.

By September 1985, I was working full-time on the newsletter, as I continue to do today. Although I didn't earn any money from the newsletter for the first few years, it pays me a salary now.

A Friend Indeed has grown primarily by word of mouth. Although we have placed small advertisements in some publications, we have found that women are more likely to trust the opinions of other women, and that the ads yield a response primarily when a woman has already heard of the newsletter elsewhere. Sometimes she may have a friend who subscribes, but often she has heard me on an open-line radio show talking about menopause. I have been the guest on so many hour-long call-in shows in all parts of North America that I am no longer surprised to pick up the telephone and hear a hesitant voice ask, "Is this the menopause lady?"

Most people assume that *A Friend Indeed* has *always* had many doctor subscribers, but we really had very few for a long time. (I am still treated with great suspicion by many physicians, perhaps because their patients tend to use me as an authority when they challenge or refuse the doctor's counsel.) But I have found that doctors' wives and nurses who work for doctors are eager to subscribe; they were the ones who put out flyers or sample issues in the doctor's waiting room! Nowadays, of course, more and more clinics and women's health centers subscribe and more and more of our flyers are finding their way into the hands of women looking for information about menopause.

When I started, I had no idea that it would take so long to achieve any level of credibility, or even that menopause was seen as the sole domain of the medical doctor. Perhaps I'm naive but I wonder why female adolescence—which represents a transitional stage between nonreproductive and reproductive status—can be discussed by psychologists, social workers, physicians, and adolescents themselves, whereas menopause—a transition between reproductive and nonreproductive status—has somehow become the bailiwick of the gynecologist? When any sort of informational meeting or presentation is planned about menopause in the United States, the organizers immediately think of inviting a gynecologist. Rarely is a menopausal woman part of the program. (And yet menopausal women are routinely invited to lecture about menopause at medical schools in other parts of the world.)

It was a shiny feather in my cap when I was asked to speak at the inaugural meetings of the North American Menopause Society (New York City, September 1989) and, even more so, when I was asked to testify about the quality of health care available to midlife women at a Congressional Subcommittee Hearing (Washington, May 1991). Since then, I have also been an invited reviewer of *Menopause, Hormone Therapy, and Women's Health*, an excellent publication issued in May 1992 by the Office of Technology Assessment, at the request of Congress.

Since 1984, I have found myself profoundly engaged in an enterprise that has been markedly different from my intended role of college teacher—which I had thought was my life's work! The success of *A Friend Indeed* is due, in large measure, to the caring and sharing of thousands of menopausal women. Through their letters, some of which are reproduced in this book, I have learned to esteem highly the knowledge and judgment of women "in the prime of life." Although the decision to invest all my energy into the newsletter meant unaccustomed isolation (me and my computer) and, at times, downright loneliness, when I do emerge from my office to travel to other cities, to speak at or to attend a conference or workshop, I am warmed by the spontaneous kindnesses and friendly hospitality I receive.

I had thought that the newsletters would suffice, but my readers persuaded me that a book—a compendium complete with index and bibliography—would be even more useful and might, in fact, be appealing to many women who are not yet *A Friend Indeed* subscribers. The Canadian version of this book was published in 1988 and continues to sell well year after year.

I am grateful to Penguin USA for the opportunity to revise and update that book for the benefit of the growing numbers of subscribers to *A Friend Indeed* in the United States, as well as for those women in their early forties who are, all unknowingly, dealing with the minor changes that precede menopause. It is my hope that the information you find here may alleviate any irrational apprehension. This book is also written for those passing through menopause. Understanding what is happening will, I think, allow you to reestablish cordial relations with a body and mind that may be temporarily out of whack, enabling you to manage your menopause with confidence.

I am grateful to my husband and my children who have put up with, and come to the aid of, a wife/mother who takes on too much, and is often too intense, too earnest, and too easily upset. When I started *A Friend Indeed* in 1984, you were all around me; we saw and touched each other every day as I revolved through the roles of mother, teacher, writer, researcher, and nag. Today, you each have your own spaces and your own loves, and I find myself transformed into, unbelievably, both doting grandmother and presiding matriarch at family get-togethers. I love each of you, just as I love the special persons you have brought into our family. And I take this opportunity to express my appreciation for your never-failing support.

I am grateful, too, to the women who have become my subscribers and my friends, and to the women who were always my friends and have now become my subscribers. You have opened my eyes to new ways of seeing this transitional period in our lives and together we are making menopause a time of life to anticipate and to relish.

REFERENCES

Budoff, P. W. *No More Menstrual Cramps and Other Good News.* NY: Penguin Books, 1981.

Cobb, J. O. *A Friend Indeed: For Women in the Prime of Life.* Box 1710, Champlain, NY 12919–1710.

Reitz, R. *Menopause: A Positive Approach.* NY: Penguin Books, 1979.

Certainly the effort to remain unchanged, young, when the body gives so impressive a signal of change as the menopause, is gallant; but it is a stupid, self-sacrificial gallantry better befitting a boy of twenty than a woman of forty-five or fifty.

—Ursula K. Le Guin, "The Space Crone,"
© 1976 by Ursula K. Le Guin;
first appeared in *CoEvolution Quarterly*.

1

How to Recognize the Onset of Menopause

Once upon a time, women were deliberately kept in ignorance of the measured steps of womanhood and the role of their own reproductive organs in menstruation, sexual intercourse, pregnancy, and menopause. Each event arrived unheralded and unknown. Today, most females in this society are encouraged to learn something about each, but the least known of them all is menopause.

During the last two or three decades, women have become conscious of entrenched sexist attitudes toward many solely female experiences—menstruation, pregnancy, childbirth. These important events in a woman's life have never been taken too seriously by the male political or medical establishments. These attitudes are changing thanks in large part to the activism of younger women. Midlife women may not be as assertive; many are faced with not only sexist attitudes but also ageist attitudes, which discount and dismiss the very real concerns of menopausal women. Rather than label ourselves as "menopausal" and thereby invite the negative stereotype of the middle-aged complainer, too many of us keep silent. And ignorance of our bodily processes feeds fear.

Isn't it strange that we would be educated in the intricacies of sexual intercourse, pregnancy, and childbirth—which are never experienced by *all women*—and yet left virtually uneducated about a process that touches *each one?* All we have to do is live long enough. These days, most women do.

> I didn't recognize the first signs of menopause. I assumed, since I was working full-time outside the home and leading a full and satisfying life, that I would be relatively untouched by it. When I finally saw a doctor about my sore wrists, I was told that it often happened "for no reason" and that there was no reliable cure. When I started feeling depressed, I assumed it was because of the constant insecurity and stress experienced by any woman in my kind of job. It got a lot worse before I belatedly recognized that menopause might be responsible.

For most of our adult lives, we are governed by cycles that are more or less predictable. Even those of us who menstruate rarely are accustomed to a predictable unpredictability of menses, or periods. The vast majority become accustomed to menstrual cycles that fall within a given time frame—always early when you don't want the bother; always late when you count on getting it over with by a certain date! By the age of twenty, most of us have learned to gauge the numbers of tampons and/or pads required and to schedule our lives around the inevitable arrival of "that time of the month." We may have even learned to laugh (in retrospect) at our excessive emotionality during the days just before menstruation. Many of us have also learned to get back into the swing after prolonged bouts of pregnancy and/or breast-feeding. The menstrual cycle is a familiar rhythm and, although we complain that it's inconvenient (or worse), we have grown accustomed to it.

This familiarity with one's own menstrual cycle is very difficult for a man to understand. Because women complain about the way menstrual cycles govern their lives, men think that we hate menstruation and want to be rid of it. Some women do. But most women learn to accommodate the vagaries of menstruation and to make allowances for it. Like an unruly pet, you complain about it but you can't imagine doing without it.

Considerable time is devoted to the accommodation of menstruation—and the time of adaptation begins even *before* menarche (the first menstrual period) when a girl's body is readying itself for the ability to menstruate. The cycle gradually regulates itself and, once established, there follows the adjustment to the physical and emotional ups and downs that occur every month. A girl who starts menstruating at about age 13 will probably take at least five years to adjust to, and be comfortable with, her own cycle and its intricate effects—emotional, psychological, and physical. Those of us who think back to our adolescence should not be surprised if, after thirty-five years, we require five years or more to readapt to *not* menstruating.

This is menopause.

If you look up the word *menopause* in a dictionary, you will not find "a five- or seven-year period marking the end of the reproductive years in women." What you *will* find is "the cessation of menstruation," a point in time that comes and goes before most of us notice.

There are some problems with this definition. First of all, naturally menopausal women can only acknowledge menopause in retrospect. We never know which menstrual period is the last until it is over. Second, there are many women who experience a last menstrual period as the result of surgical (or other artificial) interventions but who are not necessarily menopausal. An alternative, and more correct term is *climacteric*, which comes from a Greek term suggesting steps on a ladder, and which covers the whole midlife period for both males and females. Changes were thought to take place every seven years, and the odd multiples, such as thirty-five, forty-nine, and sixty-three were considered very important.

Ancient Greek society revolved around the needs and perceptions of men but, because this is a book written *by* a woman and largely *for* women, I'm going to use *menopause* in its colloquial sense: a transitional period marking the closure of reproductive life, usually (but not always) occurring during midlife. *Menopause* in this book is based on common usage—a "time of life" rather than a "point in time."

The average age at last menstrual period in America is fifty-one, but it may come earlier in some families and later in others. Any time between forty and fifty-nine falls within the realm of "normal," and each woman is undoubtedly the best judge of changes in her established pattern. Age of first menstruation seems to have very little to do with the start of menopause. Length of cycle and numbers of pregnancies may have some bearing; women who cycle every twenty-six days or so will have an earlier menopause than women who cycle every thirty-three days. Smoking will bring on an earlier menopause (up to two years earlier for a heavy smoker); and hysterectomies (removal of the uterus) and/or tubal ligations (tying or cauterization of the fallopian tubes to ensure infertility) lead to earlier menopause *in some cases*. This may be contrary to what you have been told by your doctor, but the information about hysterectomy and menopause is fairly recent: the effects of tubal ligation are strongly suspected but not yet confirmed.

Natural Menopause

A disturbance in the monthly cycle may or may not be the first sign of onset of menopause. Throughout most of our adult lives, the menstrual cycle operates in a more-or-less expected way, with hormones ebbing and flowing at levels just high enough to keep the system in comfortable balance. As you get closer to the last menstrual period, fluctuations occur—fluctuations that may affect menstruation so little as not to be noticed, but which may give you something to wonder about. Many women notice changes in bowel habits or stools; others notice headaches that come and go more frequently. There may be a difference in energy levels or the content of dreams. Many women find that their joints— knees or ankles, wrists or shoulders—start to ache for no reason. Some women experience increased premenstrual distress (PMS). Others find that they have many, very *minor* complaints when they have their regular checkups, although, paradoxically enough, life may be treating them very well in most other ways. Many women are financially more stable than in their twenties, have had time to experience the satisfactions of accomplishment, personally or professionally, and have come to terms with their physical appearance. It is only hindsight that enables many of us to recognize slight changes that occur during the early forties, changes that preceded the better-known signs of menopause.

A few years ago, I went to see my doctor regarding a pounding in my heart and aches in my joints. He never even suggested it might be menopause, stating that, at forty-two, I was too young. Thinking back, I believe it started when I was thirty-nine or forty years old. I experienced minor symptoms as early as this and am only now, at forty-four, able to recognize what these symptoms indicated.

In early puberty, anovulatory cycles (i.e., months in which no egg has been produced by the ovary) are signaled by heavier and longer bleeding than normal. In fact, many young girls have very heavy or irregular periods *until* regular ovulation is established, at which point their periods settle down to a more tolerable flow and duration. The same happens in reverse as menopause approaches. In the months

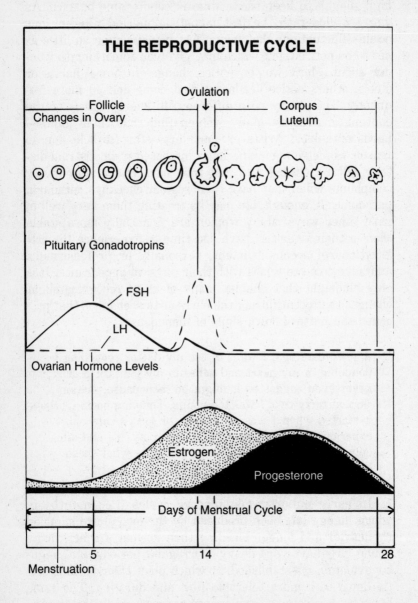

THE REPRODUCTIVE CYCLE

Ovulation

Follicle
Changes in Ovary

Corpus
Luteum

Pituitary Gonadotropins

FSH

LH

Ovarian Hormone Levels

Estrogen

Progesterone

Days of Menstrual Cycle

5   14   28

Menstruation

in which ovulation does *not* take place, periods tend to be heavier and longer. As premenopause (the time when periods are still regular) moves toward the *perimenopause* (a term used to designate the transition phase between regular periods and no periods at all), monthly events become more unpredictable. The two or three days of emotional instability that once preceded a period may escalate into a week or more of annoying and unusual premenstrual symptoms.

The onset of menopause and its accompanying ailments can be mistaken for any number of slow-acting and terminal illnesses. Unfortunately, most of us think about dying before we think of menopause, particularly when imaginations run rampant in the small hours of the morning. This tendency to view menopause as "sickness" is accentuated by our inclination to talk about menopause *symptoms*. In this book, I have tried to use less loaded terms—signs, indications, ailments. The onset of menopause is remarkable not because of any overwhelming signs that point to the end of our reproductive years, but rather because of the cumulative effect of a number of aggravating reminders that things are not as they once were.

Menopause, by itself, is rarely devastating. It is estimated that only a small minority (10 to 15 percent) of naturally menopausal women will experience severe or debilitating symptoms. Another small minority (perhaps 10 percent) will sail through with no problems whatsoever. This leaves the rest of us somewhere in the middle. Some have a rocky time but cope without drugs or other medical interventions. Others experience only infrequent and mild reminders of their menopausal status. It is the sensation of a loss of control over one's own body that is often the worst problem. If you have a reasonable idea of what to expect, managing the situation is much easier.

Artificial Menopause

There can be a significant difference between the menopause experience of a woman who has had her uterus removed (i.e., has had a hysterectomy) and a woman whose organs are intact. A substantial number of women who have had hysterectomies, *whether or not any part of the ovaries has been saved,* experience either premature menopause or a menopause quite different from that of a naturally menopausal woman. Women who have both ovaries removed (an oophorectomy or ovariectomy), or whose ovaries fail as a result of chemotherapy, will have a different kind of menopause; women who have other kinds of medical interventions (tubal ligation, complete or partial hysterectomy, radiation treatment, etc.), may not be sure whether they will have a completely natural menopause, premature menopause, or artificial menopause. (Younger women often recover from chemotherapy to resume menstruating, but women in their forties seldom do.) Rarely do physicians give their patients a clear explanation of what to expect after such intervention.

Many women are unaware of the extent of their own surgery. A *complete* hysterectomy commonly means removal of the uterus, cervix, ovaries, and fallopian tubes. But to a doctor, a complete hysterectomy means removal of the uterus and cervix only. It is important for a woman to know exactly what organs are involved in surgery if she is to understand the reasons for, and the possible consequences of, the operation.

For instance, until fairly recently, it was thought that the experience of menopause was similar for any woman who still had her ovaries or part of them—that even a small part of one ovary would continue to secrete enough estrogen to allow for menopause at the normal age. We now know that this is not true, that in many cases the remaining ovarian tissue simply cannot continue to function adequately.

The term *artificial menopause* may be applied to:

1. Those women who have had their ovaries removed (usually in conjunction with a hysterectomy).
2. Those whose ovaries fail following radiation or chemotherapy.
3. Those who experience a premature menopause as a result of a hysterectomy, even when some or all of the ovaries are untouched.

The women in categories (1) and (2) experience a very sudden menopause. The hot flashes start within a few days of surgery (or treatment) and may be brutal in their effects. At the same time, a number of other ailments may strike all at once—headaches, joint pains, fatigue, night sweats, depression, and so on. Unless there are good reasons to avoid it, estrogen therapy (ET)* is started almost immediately and may continue for some years.

The risk of depression is high for women in all three categories, with the incidence highest about two years after hysterectomy. In addition, women whose ovaries cease functioning before age forty will be at increased risk for both osteoporosis and heart disease. This is why all young women should work hard to develop bone mass, through diet and exercise, and why the experiences of natural menopause and artifical menopause should be considered separately.

Women who retain all or some of their ovaries are less severely affected. However, in from a third to a half of all cases, menopause may occur prematurely. The closer to age

---

*In cases where the ovaries have been removed or rendered inoperative, estrogen therapy is administered as estrogen *replacement* therapy (ERT). This is how any form of estrogen therapy appears in most of the literature on menopause. But ERT only "replaces" lost estrogen when it is given to women who experience an abnormal depletion of estrogen, either as a result of medical intervention or because of premature ovarian failure. Estrogen administered to women who go through natural menopause at the expected age replaces nothing, since it is perfectly normal for estrogen to be reduced at this time of life. Therefore, estrogen therapy is referred to as ET throughout this book. Similarly, hormone therapy using estrogen and progestins (synthetic progesterone) will be referred to as combined hormone therapy (CHT).

fifty at the time of the surgery, the more likely it is that
menopause will be advanced; according to recent studies,
women who are hysterectomized before the age of forty will
experience menopause an average of eight years after surgery.

> After undergoing a hysterectomy at age twenty-seven,
> I believe I am now experiencing menopause. I am
> forty-one years old. The symptoms started about four
> years ago and have included tingling sensations, anxiety,
> hot flashes, severe panic attacks, and depression. Lately
> I've been feeling so poorly that I wish I could go to
> sleep and never wake up. The three doctors I've seen
> tell me I'm too young.

Whether we experience natural or artificial menopause,
we need information beforehand and, during the period of
adjustment, most of us can use some understanding and support. To receive understanding and support, we have to be
willing to admit to our own frailties and be prepared to listen
to and affirm the experiences of other women. Unfortunately,
many women decide to unburden themselves only to one
other woman. What if (as it may turn out) this person is one
of the small minority who just stopped menstruating without
any problem? Such women often take personal credit for a
problem-free menopause (by "keeping busy," "not dwelling
on things," or "having a sense of humor"). This is not very
supportive of the woman suffering from menopausal distress!
It is then that we start asking questions: Why am I saddled
with all these problems while she gets off painlessly? Is it heredity? Is it diet? Is it the cumulative effect of medication
taken over the years? Is it the operation?
    There are no real answers to these kinds of questions.
Sisters usually have a similar experience of menopause and
go through it at roughly the same age. When there are sharp
differences, it calls into question differing experiences (diet,
exercise, sleep habits). It also highlights prior hormone use—

for adolescent acne, to induce ovulation, to prevent pregnancy, to induce delivery, to prevent miscarriage, to dry up breast milk, to alleviate hot flashes. The medical world knows very little about the effects of cumulative doses of hormones and how they might influence a woman's age at, or quality of, menopause.

Menopause and Aging

How much of a woman's experience is menopause and how much is aging? This is the million-dollar question. Because menopause and the sensation of aging often appear hand-in-hand, the careful separation of one from the other has become a matter of serious academic interest. Apparently, very few negatives can be directly attributed to menopause; depression, fatigue, anxiety, wrinkles, and gray hair are more easily linked to factors *other* than menopause. Many of the symptoms of premenstrual syndrome (PMS)—a few days of severe physical and emotional distress prior to the menstrual period—may be triggered by menopause (natural or surgical), and may continue to be felt for several years after the last menstrual period. If this is true, it means that chemical messengers in the brain produce many so-called menopausal ailments.

On the other hand, many of us know that we *have* visibly aged since our menstrual periods started to falter. Those of us who go gray in our late forties and early fifties, who find ourselves stuck with a substantial weight gain, and who also battle fatigue and aching joints, feel—not surprisingly—that menopause is responsible. In reality, it is very hard to separate aging from menopause.

It is not necessary to gain weight (although weight gain may have very positive benefits). The onset of menopause is a signal to start watching what you eat. If you feel unexpectedly tired at the end of a normal day, you would be wise to protect yourself from fatigue by cutting down on your commitments—to work, to family, to friends. Aching joints will probably disappear in time. The good news is that the menopause doldrums will pass. Once your body has adjusted to your new nonmenstruating self, you will reach a more stable and pleasant stage of development—the plateau called postmenopause.

Postmenopause is established after twelve months without a menstrual period. Margaret Mead, the famous anthropologist, introduced the term *postmenopausal zest* to describe the feelings of renewed energy and health that mark women of this age, women from their mid- to late-fifties onward. This is where one sees the sharp contrast between the listless newly retired man and his peppy, busy wife! The years after menopause are usually enormously productive.

Social Definitions of Menopause

The concept of menopause differs widely from society to society. In some societies, the onset of menopause is welcomed because it provides a break from stringent rules about what women may or may not do or say. In other societies it is regarded as an inevitable part of growing older and viewed neither positively nor negatively. In our society, which makes a fetish of both youth and slimness, menopause is often dreaded. Many of us find, much to our dismay, that we have unconsciously subscribed to our society's very narrow definition of "femininity" and that we are not willing to look our age. To deal with this, it helps to look at the social standards for men, who are often seen as *more* attractive as they age. Gray-haired and portly, their confidence projects an air of prosperity, a well-weathered masculinity. This hard-earned confidence should also be incorporated into women's views of themselves at midlife, but it often takes a conscious effort to ignore or to see beyond the stereotype of the menopausal woman and to focus on the positive aspects of the menopausal years.

This is because, in our society, a sense of loss is associated with menopause. It is not that we mourn the loss of the ability to have a baby. Most women are not interested in being a new mother at age fifty. Nor do we mourn the diminishing maternal role. Most of us are delighted to see our children step out on their own. What women mourn is the loss of their youthful image, which must now be replaced with a more mature, capable image. The mantle of middle-age descends with a thud. As Germaine Greer says:

> It isn't a gradual, imperceptible process, but happens in leaps and bounds. You can go on for years being the same age. Your face doesn't change much; your weight remains much the same. You never think of yourself as too old to learn the latest craze, can't wait to [get] off with the old and [get] on with the new. Then, crunch.
>
> You're polishing a mirror table and you realize your neck has gone. Just like that.
>
> —"Letting Go," *Vogue* magazine, May 1986, page 141

If there were an expectation of new challenges and new adventures at age fifty, menopause would be looked at much more positively. Unfortunately, in this society, the expectations and markers are almost uniformly negative. Women approach menopause with attitudes that influence how they deal with it. Because we lack positive images of women coping with menopause, the attitudes tend to be negative.

> It just seems that menopause takes over one's whole life. I was a year getting over the feelings of I-really-don't-know-what. And all of a sudden I feel "old" and realize that life is now on the down half. Immediately one is no longer young and vital—just old and tired and useless.

And yet, if we look carefully, we can find vital and healthy women in their fifties, sixties, and seventies who have overcome this negativity. Look how far we've come in relation to the women of fifty or a hundred years ago!

Confronting Menopause

Some women choose to deny the existence of menopause: this is fairly easy in our society and reflects the common attitude of dread. Unless there are definite medical reasons for not doing so, many doctors willingly prescribe estrogen (and often progesterone) so that the monthly menstrual period will continue for some years. However, this means turning a blind eye to the possible side effects and long-term consequences—in effect, abdicating the responsibility for informed choice. Women who choose to deal with menopause by avoiding it entirely are not hard to spot. Strenuous dieting, consistent application of hair color, and skillful application of makeup may minimize the effects of aging. But how long can they avoid it? What happens when time (and nature) catches up with them? How will they deal with a new "self" and an aging body—as someday we all must?

Some women give in to menopause and aging immediately. The first twinge of joint pain is interpreted as arthritis, and a sure sign of disability. Weight gain is viewed as both inevitable and an excuse for inactivity—particularly sexual activity. Anxiety and irritability are expected, often because a close friend or relative had problems at this age. With this kind of attitude, it is easy to sink into depression. As aches and pains multiply, visits to the doctor become more frequent. Because these women are the ones who turn up at doctors' offices, they too often come to personify the menopausal woman. These women are victims of our society's negative view of aging and illness, and these are the women who give menopause a bad name.

A few women will reach menopause and sail through with barely a twinge and without a backward glance. We don't know why such women are spared, although—like the research on happy marriages—it would be nice to spread the good news. The vast majority of naturally menopausal women will be bothered to some extent by minor ailments that come and go over a period of years. With some basic information about diet, exercise, and nonprescription remedies, most women can cope very well. If they are also blessed with some sincere empathy and support from friends, most women can navigate the trickier stumbling blocks of menopause.

> Regarding menopause, in all fairness to this process I must tell of spells of great well-being which come rarely, but are so strong and wonderful that I note them in my journal. They last ten to fifteen minutes and, during that time, I am totally content with the world. More than that, really: the sunshine and colors of my surroundings are perfect, my family is totally right and complete, my body and mind are just as they should be, and I am aware that all's right with the world. This is more difficult to put into words than I thought it would be. However, it is a marvelously aware and alive feeling and I think related to our time of life.
>   Yes, I have anxiety attacks and forgetfulness and mostly sleep loss, especially in the two weeks prior to my body's efforts to menstruate. My periods are getting lighter at last (I'll be fifty-three soon), but these "moments of perfection" are worth it.

The attitudes toward menopause and toward menopausal woman in *this* society have been fabricated from false assumptions, rumor, fear of aging, and media hype. Recognizing the negativism of these attitudes helps me to understand why physicians are so insistent on "treating" us, why husbands want us to take pills so we will become the wives we used to be, why younger women are apprehensive about menopause, why middle-aged women are so frightened at the prospect of aging. At the same time, I think of other societies, past and present, where midlife women are held in esteem, given special status, where they are the repositories of wisdom, the counselors of their people. This could happen again.

My hope is that, if each of us stresses the positive contributions made by the vibrant and capable midlife women in our midst (and that means you), we will change attitudes and make midlife and menopause a stage of life to be anticipated—for our daughters and, even more, our granddaughters.

REFERENCES AND RESOURCES

Backstrom, C. T., H. Boyle, and D. T. Baird. "Persistence of symptoms of premenstrual tension in hysterectomized women," *Brit. J. Obs. & Gynecol.*, *88*:530–536, May 1981.

Cattanach, J. "Oestrogen deficiency after tubal ligation," *Lancet*, *1*:847–849, April 1985.

Coulson, C. J. "Premenstrual syndrome: Are gonadotropins the cause of the condition?" *Med. Hypothesis*, *19*:243–255, 1986.

Dalton, K. *The Premenstrual Syndrome and Progesterone Therapy* (2nd ed.). Chicago: Year Book Medical Publishers, 1984.

McKinlay, S., M. Jeffreys, and B. Thompson. "An investigation of the age at menopause," *J. Biosocial. Science*, *4*:161–173, 1972.

Riedel, H-H., E. Lehmann-Willenbrock, and K. Semm. "Ovarian failure after hysterectomy," *J. Reprod. Med.*, *31*:597–600, 1986.

Siddle, N., P. Sarrel, and M. Whitehead. "The effect of hysterectomy on the age at ovarian failure: Identification of a subgroup of women with premature loss of ovarian function and literature review," *Fertil. & Steril.* *47*(1), January 1987.

2

Physical Ailments at Menopause

Sometimes it's hard to believe that women have been going through menopause for centuries. We have very little information about what the experience was like for women before us and, until someone delves into the letters and diaries of our "foremothers," we have only the misleading accounts of the men who treated them. Because there has been so little information available about menopause, we tend to view it as an impediment that must be overcome so that we can get on with our lives. This, in turn, has led to reassuring articles that tell us that we will be past it in a few months or, at most, a couple of years. The purpose is to downplay the interruption and regard adult life as a continuous line. I believe this attitude does grave disservice to the experience of menopause and its effects.

Most other animals die as soon as their reproductive lives are over. The human female is the only one to survive for such a long time after the end of her reproductive life—an average of twenty-five or thirty years, or more than a third of the lifespan. This uniquely human capacity is presumed to have evolved from the needs of the newborn human, who has an extraordinarily long dependency period, and ensures that "mother" will be on hand for the needs of the last-born. Even those who accept this as an evolutionary benefit, however, sometimes wonder why menopause operates in this way. Why does nature have to add so many hormonal upsets to the end of ovulation?

According to the theories of developmental psychology, everyone goes through stages of personality growth— periods of disruption followed by the incorporation of new learning and another step on the road to maturity. Each stage leads to new attitudes and behaviors that reflect the new learning. This is how we mature.

Most of us know something about the stages of childhood. We know that the path to maturity is marked with upheaval and that, all being well, the crises are followed by the emergence of a wiser and more self-sufficient child. The crises, of course, vary. It is hard sometimes to see the similarities between a two-year-old's tantrum, the stomachache of a seven-year-old who doesn't want to go to school, and the heartbroken sobs of a lovestruck adolescent. But the "downs" of each of these episodes are usually followed by an "up"—a painful period of self-recognition and a new stage of self-knowledge on the way to adulthood.

When we look back on our adult lives, we can often pick out similar "growth spurts"—crises faced and dealt with and new insights gained as a result. At work, these steps can be fairly easily charted. Most of us can look back at a particular rocky period that marked the taking on of more responsibility or a new level of confidence about the job. We can also see that marriage or the dissolution of marriage requires ongoing accommodation to another personality, to another situation. Out of the pain comes growth and eventually stability, either with someone else or alone. Motherhood demands new skills every few years, skills that are not easy to learn. The best mothers of babies are not always the best mothers of adolescents (which is why many of us grow nostalgic about the simpler needs of very young children). To view our own adulthood as one unbroken line that moves onward into old age is to disregard the bumpy road that we have all traveled.

One of the myths of menopause is that one enters it, weathers it, and goes back to being the same woman, only older. This is to deny the essential truth of menopause—that it is a crucial stage of development on the road to maturity, and that the experience will change us. Most women reach a new plateau of contentment *after* menopause.

In order to understand what you are (or will be) experiencing during menopause, it is important to recognize a range of symptoms—both physical and psychological—that commonly affect women during this time. Although it's almost certain that you will not experience more than a few of these ailments, it helps to have heard about them just in case you *do* experience them.

Despite the documented occurrence of all of the ailments listed, most medical texts recognize only three major physical ailments—menstrual irregularity, hot flashes, and dry vagina (or genito-urinary distress). Osteoporosis is occasionally listed as a symptom of menopause but it is, in fact, a condition that begins long before menopause but which may become critical during the menopausal years. Psychological ailments (anxiety, panic attacks, and depression) are viewed in very different ways, depending on the source or the expert you consult. The three major physical ailments (sometimes expanded to four with the addition of osteoporosis) that follow are the ones that most doctors are prepared to discuss and treat.

MENOPAUSAL AILMENTS

Menstrual irregularity
⚹ Hot flashes and/or flushes; night sweats
Dry vagina
⚹ Insomnia and/or weird dreams
Sensory disturbances (vision, smell, alterations to taste)
Funny sensations in the head
Lower back pain (crushing of vertebrae)
Waking in the early hours of the morning
Onset of new allergies or sensitivities
Fluctuations in sexual desire and sexual response
Annoying itching of the vulva (area around vagina)
Sudden bouts of bloat (waistline expands by two to three inches
    for an hour or two)
Chills or periods of extreme warmth
Indigestion, flatulence, gas pains
Rogue chin whiskers
Overnight appearance of long, fine facial hairs
⚹ Bouts of rapid heartbeat
Crying for no reason
Aching ankles, knees, wrists, or shoulders
Waking up with sore heels
Thinning scalp and underarm hair
Graying scalp and pubic hair
Mysterious appearance of bruises
Sudden inability to breathe ("air hunger")
Frequent urination
Urinary leakage (when coughing or sneezing, or during orgasm)
Prickly or tingly hands with swollen veins
Lightheadedness, dizzy spells, or vertigo
Weight gain and in unusual places (on the back, breasts, abdomen)
Sudden and inappropriate bursts of anger
Sensitivity to touching by others ("touch impairment")
Inexplicable panic attacks
Tendency to cystitis (inflammation of the bladder)
Vaginal or urethral infections
Anxiety and loss of self-confidence
⚹ Depression that cannot be shaken off
Painful intercourse
Migraine headaches
Easily wounded feelings
Crawly skin ("formication")
Disturbing memory lapses

Standard Signs of Menopause

Menstrual Irregularity

The most common sign of menopause is a fluctuation in the menstrual cycle. Although this may not be the *first* indication of menopausal onset, it is the one most women look for. Periods may continue to arrive on time, but there are often minor changes. The woman who once could relax for an hour or two between the first "show" and the need for a pad or tampon may find that she is now very quickly staining her clothes. The period that lasted three or four days may last for two or for six. The color of the flow may change—rather than moving from red to brown, it may be brown then redder, then brown again. All of this is normal, as is the increasing tendency to skip a period now and then, or to have two or three periods back to back. If you are familiar with your own rhythm, you will be more exasperated by all this than alarmed.

The cessation of my menstrual periods was gradual. It lasted for approximately three years, and the uncertainty was most irritating and often quite embarrassing. I experienced minor symptoms of menopause, such as lightheadedness and hot flashes, during this time. However, now that my periods have ceased altogether, menopause has arrived in full force. I am experiencing hot flashes, mood swings, and dry vagina. I realize now that it is specifically during the first signs of menopause— that is, erratic menses—that one should take the opportunity to inform oneself fully about the years to follow.

What is *not* normal is bleeding between periods. If you experience this, be sure to consult your doctor.

Hot Flashes and Night Sweats

Another very common physical symptom is the hot flash. In North America, we say "flash"; in England, it is commonly "flush." But they are not necessarily the same thing. A hot flash is the sudden sensation of heat (it may be experienced as a result of stress in the absence of menopause). A hot flush is the red neck or face that is visible to others. (You may have a red chest or back as well.) You can have a flush without feeling a flash, and you can feel a flash without "giving it away" with a flush. Hot flashes experienced during the night are called night sweats. Some women experience flashes but no night sweats; some experience only night sweats; some experience both. And some women don't have hot flashes; they have cold chills, which is just a variation.

The onset of hot flashes is often heralded by the unexpected return of the old-fashioned "blush." Many women find their faces reddening without feeling any sensation of warmth. The first experience of a hot flash may be nothing more than a feeling of unusual warmth; you may throw the covers off, or remove a jacket or sweater and not think about it further. It is estimated that between 75 to 85 percent of American women experience hot flashes—some for only a few weeks and some for as long as fifteen to twenty years. And the real thing is unmistakable. Many women are aware of it before it even starts, with feelings ranging from slight nausea to a sense of doom: "Something terrible is about to happen!" In studies done of hot flashes, women are often able to say, "Here comes one!" before the medical instruments start to show any differences in skin temperature or blood circulation. After the "advance signal" there may be a rapid buildup—often concentrated in the chest and upper body—followed by a rise in body temperature and a feeling of unbearable heat. The veins of the hands may tingle and swell. Perspiration may bead at the hairline, between the breasts, down the back. Hot flashes can last from one minute to one hour, but most are over in two to three minutes.

There may be a chilly sensation for a few moments afterward.

> I would like every man and woman to have just one of *my* hot flashes! First, a sudden, unexplained what's-the-point-of-it-all feeling which lasts only five or ten seconds. I know that, within the next thirty seconds, I'm going to have a hot flash—waves of heat traveling up my body, perspiration breaking out all over and running down my forehead, a terrible feeling of weakness and exhaustion. I have to sit down or lean against a wall if no seats are available. I'm left with damp clothes (which quickly start to feel cold) and I feel as if I've just finished a hard game of squash—a game I had to give up some years ago. Sometimes I can feel my head pounding during the flash, and sometimes it leaves me with a headache. This can happen from once an hour to four or five times in an hour.

Hot flashes tend to appear during the time when menstrual periods are erratic and to peak during the year of the last menstrual period. They seem to occur most often just before rising and just before bed (six a.m. and ten p.m.) and, although many women believe that stress makes the flashes worse, some women find that the frequency and intensity are *not* affected by unusual stress or worry. Such women report equally heavy flashing during times of rest or relaxation with friends.

The nighttime version of the hot flash is usually more severe. Perspiration may be so profuse as to require a change of clothing or of bed linen. Night sweats that are severe and/or frequent contribute to fatigue and depression. Fortunately, most naturally menopausal women rarely experience flashes this severe.

Dry Vagina and Urinary Distress

With the onset of menopause, there is a tendency for the tissue of the urethra and vagina to thin out and become more fragile. The vagina may also become shorter and both urethra and vagina become more vulnerable to inflammation and infection. Dry vagina (also known by the medical, but offensive-to-women term, *senile vaginitis*) may mean that a woman's own lubrication is inadequate for pleasurable penile penetration. In extreme cases, the vagina may be so dry as to make routine movements like walking uncomfortable. This condition is likely to occur a few years after menopause (i.e., usually during the late fifties or early sixties) or as a result of artificial menopause (involving removal of the ovaries).

Recurring cystitis (a burning sensation when urinating) or other urinary problems may occur after hysterectomy as a result of surgery, rather than from natural aging. Damage to the bladder or ureters (tubes running from the bladder to the kidneys) is not uncommon following this operation, particularly if the procedure was done through the vagina—as, for instance, to repair a prolapse.

Even when vaginal or urinary problems are relatively minor, many women complain of frequent urination and a tendency to "leak" when coughing, sneezing, or during orgasm. This is known as *stress incontinence. Urge incontinence* is diagnosed when urine is dribbled on the way to the toilet. Both complaints are common and both are eminently treatable.

Osteoporosis

Osteoporosis means "porous bone" and is a condition that results from excess loss of bone tissue. The onset of osteoporosis is usually painless (which is why it is not listed as a menopausal ailment) and osteoporotic women rarely get advance warning of its onset, except for periodic backache (often of the lower back) as crush fractures occur. Because the pain eases after a few days and then goes away, few women suspect that a vertebra has collapsed. For most women, the first awareness of osteoporosis follows from a broken bone, often a wrist fracture. This fracture may lead to a series of fractures.

Strictly speaking, osteoporosis is *not* a symptom of menopause, because its onset is based on many factors in addition to menopausal status, and most particularly on bone density at about age thirty-five—long before menopause starts. Bone continues to strengthen (i.e., become more dense) until the mid-thirties after which we start to lose bone—at first slowly and then more quickly as we reach the late forties and early fifties. Once menopause is past, bone loss slows down again.

It is suspected that osteoporosis may comprise a number of different conditions and there is still a great deal to be known about it. We *do* know, however, that there are at least two types of bone involved—cortical (the hard, shiny outer layer) and trabecular (the honeycomb structure of inner bone or vertebrae). Each type of bone may be affected by a number of factors and, unless you have worked hard to build strong bones during your young adulthood (i.e., consumed a lot of calcium and had regular vigorous exercise), you may have grounds for concern. If you are slight, fair-skinned, if you smoke, do not exercise regularly, have never borne or breast-fed a child, and have a history of broken bones in your family, you should take steps to prevent excess loss of bone.

Aside from menstrual irregularity, hot flashes, dry vagina, and osteoporosis, a number of ailments, minor and major, are everyday occurrences for many menopausal women. What such complaints have in common is that they are only rarely blamed on menopause, whether in books or articles, or in the opinions of most medical practitioners. Indeed, it is sometimes difficult to know whether they are caused by menopause or by aging—a situation that is likely to persist until more solid research is available.

Other Complaints

If you mention one of these "additional" ailments to your doctor, you are likely to have it dismissed. It very much depends on the person you consult. A knowledgeable physician may take some of these ailments seriously, but it is hard to know which complaint will be attended to and which will be trivialized.

Joint Pains

This common ailment often appears before either menstrual irregularity or the first hot flash. When bursitis of the shoulder, tennis elbow, trick knees, aching wrists, sore heels, or "funny" ankles occur, menopause is rarely suspected; but joint aches appear to be linked to the adrenal glands where cortisone (the substance that keeps joints moving freely) is manufactured. Studies have shown that from one-fifth to one-half of menopausal women experience joint pain at one time or another. It appears to afflict women of all sizes and shapes, whether they engage in regular, vigorous exercise or are somewhat sedentary.

Joint pain is usually restricted to one or two joints, and should not be considered in the same class as chronic aches and pains, which may recur for years. Chronic and severe aches and pains may be due to fibromyalgia (explained in detail in Vol. VII, No. 9 of *A Friend Indeed*). Women with fibromyalgia are often mistakenly diagnosed as either arthritic or osteoporotic although there is no muscle inflammation, damaged tissue, swollen joints, or broken bones. Women who have had a hysterectomy appear more vulnerable to fibromyalgia, but this is still under investigation. It is not likely to happen to you, but those women who have exhausted every other possibility in the search for an explanation for massive aches and pains should know about fibromyalgia.

Migraine

Migraine headaches begin with a spasm in an artery close
to the surface, on either the left or right side of the head.
Because the headache is confined to one side of the head,
a migraine is quite different from a stress headache (which
usually comes on slowly) or the "hatband" sensation of a
tension headache. Some women will experience bouts of dizziness, strange tingling sensations, or episodes of rapid
heartbeat ("palpitations"); these may be forms of migraine
activity *without* the headache. Some women will notice
strange "pings" in the back of the head, or what feel like
strange surges of blood. It is wise to check out any such
symptoms with a doctor, even though these experiences are
fairly common.

I experienced severe attacks of vertigo intermittently
over a one-year period and they only stopped after
a self-imposed regimen of vitamin supplements—
vitamin B_{12}, vitamin C, and a multiple vitamin tablet.
The attacks usually came on when I got out of my car
in the company parking lot to walk the 150 feet to
the entrance. During an attack, if I got up from my
chair too quickly, I felt as if I would fall over and, while
walking the hallways, I would literally bump into the
walls. Now that it is over, I can only attribute the
spells of vertigo to stressful situations.

The relationship between migraines and hormones has
been inferred from the onset of common migraine at puberty,
the cyclical nature of the symptoms, and the tendency for migraines to disappear (in about 80 percent of cases) during
pregnancy, and to return again until postmenopause when,
in the majority of cases, they disappear for good.

Some women, however, develop migraines for the first
time just prior to menopause. The migraines, whether in the
form of headaches or not, occur most commonly during the

menstrual period or in the few days following the period. The timing is assumed to be related to low levels of progesterone, but other patterns—headache at ovulation, or just prior to menstruation—may be related to estrogen levels. Or it may be the ratio of estrogen to progesterone that triggers the migraine.

Some women will experience the typical aura (or *prodrome)* that precedes a migraine without ever having the headache. The aura is a subjective sensation, warning that a migraine is about to start. The aura may take many forms—dizziness, numbness, tingling of the extremities, heightened sensitivity to smells or noise or taste, restlessness, yawning, and so on—but the more common aura is a visual disturbance marked by spots floating before the eyes, then a shimmering outline that gradually obliterates most of the visual field.

Other migraine equivalents are abdominal pain with nausea, vomiting, or diarrhea; acute pain in the chest, pelvis, or extremities; attacks of rapid heartbeat (tachycardia); sudden attacks of dizziness for no apparent reason (benign paroxysmal vertigo); or bloat occurring on a cyclical basis—repeated after a predictable number of days. Each of these symptoms may or may not be accompanied by a headache.

There is no one simple test to establish the presence of a migraine and, even less so, of a migraine equivalent. If you suspect that you are experiencing a migraine equivalent, you might ask your doctor to arrange for medical tests to rule out other possibilities. (Inner-ear infections, for example, could be responsible for the dizziness.) Or you may wish to see a neurologist who specializes in migraine.

Burning Mouth Syndrome

Some women experience dry mouth during menopause, a condition that is often aggravated by caffeine and antihistamines, as well as some prescription drugs (e.g., clonidine and some kinds of antidepressants). Because oral tissue is structurally similar to vaginal tissue, dry mouth is thought to be related to the more widely recognized problem of dry vagina. (If dry mouth is accompanied by dry eyes, you should look into the possibility of Sjögren's syndrome.) Others suffer from an extreme case of dry mouth, called burning mouth syndrome (BMS) estimated to affect only 2 percent of the general population, of whom as many as one-fifth may be postmenopausal women. Burning mouth syndrome often prompts a visit to the dentist with complaints about a chronically burning sensation in the mouth and gums, but the cause is not yet understood.

Indigestion, Flatulence, Bloat

Many women complain about indigestion or flatulence. Some also occasionally experience "bloat"—the lower torso (waist and belly) swells and remains swollen for two or three hours. This is a very uncomfortable feeling, one that many women remember from pregnancy!

Sleep Problems

Changes in sleep habits are very common. Many women find it hard to get to sleep, to stay asleep, or to sleep past the light of early dawn. The average number of hours spent sleeping diminishes from about eight hours at age twenty to about six hours at age fifty, and there is a concurrent increase in awakenings. Some of this sleeplessness may be due to hot flashes which, although not severe enough to warrant the term *night sweats*, are enough to waken. Once wakened, many of us head for the toilet. It's hard to know what provokes the wakening—the sensation of warmth or a full bladder.

Most physicians assume that hot flashes cause sleep disruption and that the alleviation of the flashes (using estrogen) will result in restful sleep. Sometimes this is true, but some women experience severe sleep problems that cannot be remedied with estrogen therapy (ET).

Menopause may also be marked by episodes of "air hunger," a sudden and unpleasant sensation of suffocation—gasping for air for a few minutes until it passes. A variation is *sleep apnea*, where breathing stops for a few interminable seconds. Although both sensations last for only a short time, they can be very frightening.

> I have had several unpleasant episodes of sleep apnea over the last two years, two of them severe enough to warrant hospitalization. I really felt quite crazy when I was explaining that I had stopped breathing for a few seconds, but a friend who accompanied the recent Everest expedition had similar symptoms due to the altitude. Unfortunately, my doctor can't offer any help or explanation for this distressing complaint. Neurological tests show nothing wrong.

Weight Gain

This is not, strictly speaking, an ailment because it is so widespread. However, many of us find ourselves being chided by our doctors and this, together with our own futile efforts to slim, make it *feel* like a medical problem. Most of us do not eat more than usual. The weight gain is a feature of aging, but is hastened by menopause, when the metabolism slows down. Not only are the extra pounds both unexpected and unwelcome, but they often accumulate in strange places—on the back, bust, and abdomen—rather than on the hips and thighs.

Skin and Hair

Some women complain of a crawling sensation on the skin. The proper medical term for this is *formication*, which is related to *formicary*, an ant nest. It feels as if small ants are crawling on the skin. Patterns of hair growth may change, with underarm hair, pubic hair, and scalp hair thinning out and changing texture, while unwanted facial hair makes an appearance. If scalp hair is thinning (frontal hair loss), a dermatologist or endocrinologist may be needed. The cause is usually assumed to be hereditary male-pattern baldness emerging as the male hormones (androgens) assume more importance in our bodies.

I am taking estrogen and, so far, have had no problems with it. However, my unhappiness now—and yes, I can call it that—is that my hair, once curly and pretty, is thinning *drastically*. Of course, I have changed my hairstyle and tried various "cosmetics" for hair to keep it up and back. I try to ignore the situation, but am privately terrified. I'm fifty-four years old and want to continue my busy, productive life without the threat of a wig!

Frontal hair loss may also result, paradoxically, from an excess of estrogen—either manufactured in the body (most often by obese women) or taken as estrogen supplements. If scalp hair is thinning too rapidly and in patches, the condition may be alopecia areata, which is not related to menopause.

Sensory Disturbances

Many women experience what are known as sensory disturbances during menopause, either briefly or for a more extended period of time. They may feel their vision worsening

and need a new eyeglass prescription, or they may merely
see spots in front of their eyes now and then. Some women
report that they hear bursts of sounds more loudly than
usual. Some women smell phantom aromas for weeks or
months at a time—woodsmoke, wet grass, or a dimly remembered scent impossible to identify. Some develop a sensitivity
to certain tastes, or lose the sense of taste almost entirely.
(This latter condition may also be due to use of corticosteroids.) Some women experience *touch impairment*, a sensitivity to being touched which makes them jumpy, "touchy,"
unable to respond to previously welcome touching by others.
These conditions are usually temporary.

Other Problems

In addition, there are a potpourri of annoying physical
changes, some of which may be linked to menopause (such as
swollen, tender breasts) but most of which may be due to aging. Many women feel overwhelming fatigue, probably due to
the sheer stress of all the internal bodily changes occurring,
but sometimes worsened by interrupted sleep (although one
is not necessarily conscious of the interruptions), or thyroid
underactivity (hypothyroidism). Some women get "rubber
legs," the temporary but frightening sensation that their legs
are going to give way underneath them. Some notice weird
bruises. It has even been reported that, because of hormonal
changes, menopausal women are more likely to suffer from
bad breath!

There is no way of predicting who will experience what
ailments, who will have a tough time, and who will have an
easy time. Nor is there any magic formula to determine who
can and cannot cope. The experience of menopause is as individual as the experiences of pregnancy or childbirth.

If your ailments are more of a nuisance than anything
else, you can probably deal with them on your own. Many of

the physical ailments of menopause can be managed by alterations in daily routines to eliminate bad habits (smoking and caffeine), to include regular exercise, to add key nutrients to the diet, or to cut back on commitments in order to relieve the stress on your system. Because your immediate interest is in resuming a regular routine, the knowledge that these ailments are likely to be temporary and that they are experienced by many menopausal women will help to restore a sense of control. From this control comes the confidence necessary to deal with the temporary inconveniences of the menopausal years.

If you are feeling ill and unable to deal with day-to-day responsibilities, you should seek professional help. Unfortunately, many doctors do not relate menopause to many of these ailments and, if they do, often do not share this information with their patients. The attitude seems to be that menopausal women are eager to complain, and ready to "adopt an ailment" and call it their own. If your ailments are medical, you will need a good physician. More and more doctors are learning to be sympathetic and helpful to their menopausal patients. Shop around for this type of doctor. If your menopausal ailments derive from poor nutrition or poor general health, or if they affect your relationships, you may want to consult a holistic health practitioner, a naturopath, a counselor, or a psychotherapist. If you are fortunate, you will find a professional who will work *with* you to find answers to your questions and relief from the most worrisome complaints.

REFERENCES AND RESOURCES

Ballinger, S. E. "A comparison of life stresses and symptomatology of menopause clinic patients and non-patients." Paper presented at the 4th International Congress on the Menopause, Buena Vista, Florida, 1984.

Cobb, J. O. "Fibromyalgia: The sore-all-over syndrome." *A Friend Indeed.* 7(9), February, 1991.

Dudley, R. and W. Rowland. *How to Find Relief from Migraine*. Toronto: Collins, 1982.

Feldman, B. M., A. Voda, and E. Gronseth. "The prevalence of hot flash and associated variables among perimenopausal women," *Res. Nursing & Health*, *8*:261–268, 1985.

Gillespie, L. *You Don't Have to Live with Cystitis*. NY: Rawson Associates, 1987.

Grushka, M., B. J. Sessle, and R. Miller. "Pain and personality profiles in Burning Mouth Syndrome", *J. Pain*, *28*(2):155–167, February 1987.

"Hair, beautiful hair," U. of Toronto Faculty of Medicine *Health News*, *6*(4):1–5, August 1988.

Kronenberg, F., L. J. Cote, and D. M. Linkie. "Menopausal hot flashes: Thermoregulatory, cardiovascular and circulating catecholamine and LH changes," *Maturitas*, *6*(1):31–43, 1984.

Notelovitz, M. and M. Ware. *Stand Tall: The Informed Woman's Guide to Preventing Osteoporosis*. Florida: Triad Publishing, 1982.

Price, V. H. "Women and hair loss: Alopecia areata," *National Women's Health Report*, *3*(5), May 1985.

Sacks, O. *Migraine: Evolution of a Common Disorder*. London, Faber & Faber, 1970.

Voda, A. M. "Menopausal hot flash," *Changing Perspectives on Menopause*, Voda et al., eds. Austin: U. of Texas Press, 1982.

Voda, A. M., B. M. Feldman, and E. Gronseth. "Description of the hot flash: sensations, meaning and change in frequency across time." Paper presented at the 4th International Congress on the Menopause, Buena Vista, Florida, 1984.

Woods, N. F. "Menopausal distress: A model for epidemiological investigation," in *Changing Perspectives on Menopause*, Voda et al., eds. Austin: U. of Texas Press, 1982.

3

Strategies and Remedies:
Medical and Nonmedical

The decision to seek medical help is often a difficult one. Because menopause has never been a major part of medical studies, many physicians haven't learned much about it, have not taken it seriously and, rather than listening to their patients, have simply told them to keep busy or to stop thinking about themselves. At the other extreme, gynecologists—the specialists who are *expected* to know about menopause—are often so occupied with women who are truly ill (primarily those who have been hysterectomized), that they view menopause as worse than it really is. Only a few naturally menopausal women have a dreadful time but, because the medical view of menopause defines it as a disease rather than as a normal transition, a specialist may be *too* willing to prescribe powerful drugs.

According to many textbooks on menopause, there are three "symptoms" of menopausal onset: menstrual irregularity, hot flashes, and dry vagina. This is what most doctors look for when you mention menopause. They may also discuss osteoporosis, although osteoporosis is *not* a menopausal complaint because it is waiting in the wings long before menopause arrives (see Chapter 6). But most doctors won't discuss a list of menopausal ailments about which women complain to each other (and to *me*), and which are rarely covered in the medical literature. These are covered in the second part of this chapter.

If you view menopause as a natural transition (as I do), you may be interested in ways to make menopause as smooth as possible, including preventive steps and nonmedical ("alternative") remedies. Many women never think of going to a naturopath, nutritionist, chiropractor, or acupuncturist, despite the fact that they have helped many menopausal women. Perhaps the fundamental need is a basic interest in the problem. If you are willing to try readily available remedies, you may be able to manage your own menopause without resorting to prescribed medication. Be aware, however, that nonmedical remedies often do not provide immediate relief. The benefits of regular exercise, vitamin or diet supplements, not smoking, and such do not appear overnight. If you decide to experiment with an alternative remedy, be patient. Give each product a fair trial—at least a month or two—before abandoning it. Because more is not necessarily better, it is dangerous to take more than the recommended amounts. If you do your shopping in health food stores, you may find leaflets and publications that often make extravagant claims for various products. Be wary of farfetched claims made by some manufacturers or packagers. Alternative remedies are not enforced as strictly as prescription drugs.

Menstrual Irregularity

Before you make an appointment with your doctor, it is wise to jot down exactly what is bothering you. If it is menstrual irregularity, keep track of your periods for a few months. Write down the frequency and duration of each period as well as lightness/heaviness and color of the flow. Because ovulation takes place less and less frequently as we approach menopause, progesterone is sometimes not produced. Because progesterone induces menstruation, cycles without progesterone are often later with heavier and more profuse bleeding. Cycles that produce such erratic and heavy bleeding can be very bothersome, so it is reassuring to know that this is often a temporary situation preceding true menopause.

Nonprescription Remedies

Some women have found relief from a heavy flow by taking vitamin A supplements (10,000 IU, or International Units, twice daily), by taking over-the-counter antihistamines, or by using a painkiller such as ibuprofen. A controlled study in Britain found that acupuncture often relieves heavy bleeding.

Many women have avoided minor surgery by keeping records. One woman told me that she had not menstruated for three months. She then had a prolonged period (fifteen days of heavy flow), which might have warranted further investigation. However, her notes on the color and consistency of the flow established that this was actually three periods back to back.

Keep track of when and where you experience any unusual symptoms. Did something happen beforehand that might account for it? Have you had similar experiences in the past?

Medical Interventions

Bleeding may sometimes be controlled using naproxen, a mild antiinflammatory often prescribed for menstrual cramps, or a low-dose contraceptive pill. Although oral contraceptives have been considered inadvisable for women over forty, the new low-dose pills do not pose the same kinds of problems in terms of potential cardiovascular risk. To be on the safe side, however, it is better to quit smoking before taking "the pill."

An alternative to the pill is progesterone therapy, sometimes called a *medical D&C*. Synthetic progesterone (usually Provera at 10 mg or 5 mg daily) is administered for ten days; two days later a normal bleed takes place. This therapy can be continued for months until the bleed is negligible, at which point it is inferred that very little estrogen is being produced by the ovaries.

If neither the pill nor the progesterone therapy is effective, a D&C (dilatation and curettage) may be advised. This procedure often corrects heavy bleeding due to polyps or some forms of uterine fibroids. And newer procedures, which employ a hysteroscope (a fiber-optic device enabling the surgeon to see into the uterus), together with a tiny instrument that fits inside the hysteroscope, permit the doctor to scrape or burn away the lining of the uterus (and the small fibroids that it may conceal). This means sacrificing fertility, but it is a minor procedure compared to a hysterectomy and it doesn't entail the aftereffects of major surgery.

Hot Flashes and Night Sweats

If you experience hot flashes, write down the dates, times, and duration of each. If you suspect that certain "triggers" bring on a hot flash, keep track. You may find that you can eliminate or manage heavy flashing by giving up caffeine, reducing or eliminating alcohol and certain foods or activities, and choosing different activities at times of day that seem to bring them on. Some women find that they can quickly ward off a hot flash by drinking iced water or by splashing the face with cold water. And, of course, you will find it easier to cope if you dress in layers and wear natural fibers that breathe, rather than synthetics.

One of the least known but most effective ways of minimizing hot flashes is to gain weight. The discomforts that accompany menopause are, to a large degree, caused by the erratic and diminishing production of estradiol (a form of estrogen) by the ovaries, and the shift to estrone, an alternative and less powerful form of estrogen. It is useful to know that menopause is *not* the end of estrogen production but rather a time when the body "shifts gears" and begins to utilize estrogen of a different kind at a different level. Some ovaries continue to produce estradiol fitfully but successfully for months or even years. At the same time, androstenedione, a substance produced by both the ovaries and the adrenal glands, is being converted into estrone (a secondary form of estrogen) in the adipose (or fatty) tissue of the body. This conversion process becomes more efficient and more effective with age and with a healthy ratio of body fat.

To encourage this shift to estrone production, many nutritionists and geriatricians encourage menopausal women to tolerate a gain of ten to fifteen pounds over "ideal weight." The added weight is also helpful in combating osteoporosis. So don't get *too* upset if a few extra pounds manage to slip onto your frame. The slender women you have always envied may be more affected by hot flashes and may also be more prone to broken bones in old age.

Nonprescription Remedies

The most popular products to combat hot flashes are vitamins E and C, evening primrose oil (often recommended for premenstrual syndrome), bee pollen, ginseng, and dong quai.

Vitamin E is measured in International Units (100, 200, 400, etc.); the bottled capsules are available in drugstores and health food stores. Vitamin E is reputed to be effective for one-half to two-thirds of women with hot flashes, but it may take from two to six weeks to notice the difference. Women with diabetes, high blood pressure, or a rheumatic heart condition should only take very small quantities, a maximum of 100 International Units daily. *Vitamin E should not be taken by someone on digitalis.* Most women will be comfortable with 600 to 800 IU, preferably taken after a meal containing some fat. Some advocates of vitamin E recommend that it be taken with vitamin C.

Another popular supplement to combat infection and to counteract the effects of environmental pollution, vitamin C is measured in grams and is usually recommended in doses of no more than one gram (1000 mg) a day, and 500 mg may be sufficient. Too much vitamin C may cause diarrhea or stomach upset. (Chewable vitamin C is bad for the teeth.) To make both vitamin E and vitamin C more accessible to the body, it is recommended that selenium (25 mcg for each 200 IU of E) and bioflavinoids (100 mg for each 500 mg of C) be added.

If you are unsure of the types and amounts of diet supplements that might help your particular situation, you may want to consult a nutritionist, a naturopath, or a doctor versed in holistic medicine. If you don't know whom to consult, check with your local health food store to see if they can recommend someone. You can also find the names and addresses in the Yellow Pages, or in the directories printed in many "alternative" magazines on the newsstand.

Evening primrose oil (EPO) is another popular remedy for hot flashes. EPO contains gamma-linolenic acid, which is related to prostaglandin activity, fatty acids involved in the contraction of blood vessels. Evening primrose oil is promoted for relief of menstrual cramps, swollen and tender breasts, and hot flashes. Be sure that the product you choose contains a significant amount of gamma-linolenic acid (40 to 50 percent), because there are some very poor-quality products on the market. Good EPO is expensive, but women who use it regularly (for both PMS and menopause symptoms) swear by it, although there are as yet no reputable studies establishing its effectiveness. The recommended dose is two to eight capsules daily. Other sources for gamma-linolenic acid are borage oil and spirulina (blue-green algae).

Bee pollen, like evening primrose oil, has been popularized through the menopause grapevine. Various products have been recommended to me, some in the form of pleasantly chewable tablets at a recommended dose of one a day. These products may also be expensive.

Ginseng and dong quai (or tan kwai—the spelling varies) are herbs originally imported from the Orient, although most ginseng is now grown here. The ginseng root *(panax ginseng* or *panax quinquefolius)* is recommended for both men and women as a way of increasing the metabolic rate and regaining energy. Ginseng is processed as tablets, capsules, liquid, powder, or tea. People with asthma or emphysema are advised to avoid it because of its histamine-liberating action. Dong quai (angelica sinensis) is often sold as "female ginseng" and is said to have hormonelike properties capable of relieving severe hot flashes. I have found it in tablets and powders. (It is interesting to note that, in China, the use of such herbs and preparations is supervised by pharmacists who spend six years learning their profession. Medical doctors in China go to school for only five years.)

A few years ago, I first become aware of occasionally feeling hot all by myself; no one else seemed to find it too warm. I remember a summer holiday, a 300-mile drive with all the car windows open; I was dressed in two layers of batiste cotton and my torso was sheeted with pouring sweat. I had neglected to renew my supply of ginseng about a week before the trip.

My experience was that, so long as I kept ginseng and vitamin E as part of my morning regimen, I experienced no hot flashes nor any other discomfort. The whole business was over in three years with not a ripple of reminder since.

Ginseng is also considered to have estrogenic properties, which means that moderation should be the rule. Other sources of estrogen-like substances are to be found in red clover sprouts, linseed, and soy flour. Diets high in any of these foods will produce a measurable biological response—and may also alleviate hot flashes.

Prescription Remedies

Clonidine is the generic name of a hypertensive drug (commonly prescribed as Catapres adhesive patches), which is sometimes successful in controlling hot flashes. Because clonidine may contribute to depression, avoid it if you have depressive tendencies. It appears to be more effective if started before flashes become really severe. Even so, it works for only 30 to 40 percent of the women who try it. The patches are available in doses of .1 mg, .2 mg, and .3 mg, and are usually applied once a week. You should feel a difference within two to three weeks if it's going to work. Potential side effects are dry mouth, constipation, headaches and, occasionally, wild dreams. It is recommended that medication be discontinued, but always very slowly, after three to six months, for reevaluation of the situation.

Bellergal is another drug occasionally prescribed for hot flashes. A third of the women who try this medication suffer an adverse reaction and must discontinue it. Even when it does work, you should know that Bellergal contains belladonna, phenobarbitol, and ergotamine tartrate, and is potentially addictive. For this reason, most health activists feel that it is not suitable for the treatment of menopause.

Occasionally prescribed—for women who cannot or will not take estrogen—are propranolol (Inderal), a beta-blocker, the antihypertensive, methyldopa (Aldomet), and the dopamine agonist, bromocriptine (Parlodel), or a progestin (Provera). In Europe, a number of studies have been published using veralipride, an anti-dopaminergic compound that has been 60 to 80 percent successful in reducing hot flashes. Little interest has been shown in this alternative in this country.

There are many estrogen products available, but dominating the U.S. market is Premarin, a tablet or pill taken once daily (see chapter 5). Second only to Premarin is the Estraderm patch, which is applied twice a week to the thigh, bottom, or abdomen.

Either product offers speedy relief of debilitating hot flashes. Although it will not eliminate *all* flashes for *all* women, it is the most effective prescription remedy available. Because the decision about whether to seek or to accept estrogen therapy (ET) remains the central issue for many menopausal women, additional information on the use of ET and CHT (Combined Hormone Therapy) is outlined in Chapter 5.

If you are considering use of hormone therapy primarily to relieve hot flashes, you may want to know that:

- Hot flashes last longer for women on hormone therapy.
- Although hot flashes may be alleviated while on hormones, there is a strong possibility that the flashes may return with a vengeance as soon as therapy is discontinued. In other words, hormone therapy masks or postpones hot flashes rather than eliminating them entirely.
- There are specific contraindications to hormone therapy (reasons why some women cannot or should not take hormones). You should be aware of these in case your doctor is not (see chapter 5).
- There are potential side effects to estrogen and synthetic progesterones (as there are to any drug). You should know what they are so that you can recognize and deal with them in case they arise.
- Many physicians have personal preferences based on limited experience with certain forms, methods of administration, and dosages (i.e., regimens) of hormone therapy. If you are unhappy with your regimen, you

have the right to insist on something different until you find what is appropriate for your unique chemistry.

It is hysterectomized and, most of all, oophorectomized women who suffer from the most severe hot flashes. For these women, and for the small minority of naturally menopausal women who find their hot flashes intolerable, estrogen provides the only certain relief. Most naturally menopausal women suffer as much or more from fatigue due to the physiological stress of constantly adjusting to internal temperature changes, and to the embarrassment at having a hot flash in public. If the social stigma of this kind of "flashing" were removed and the embarrassment eliminated, we would all feel better. As more and more women experience the novelty of the hot flash, the day may come when menopausal women will feel free to have hot flashes anywhere, without censure, without shame.

Dry Vagina, Cystitis, Vaginitis

Naturally menopausal women may notice changes in the frequency and pattern of urination while still menstruating, and hysterectomized women may experience urinary distress at an even earlier age. This is often caused by damage to the bladder or ureters during surgery, particularly vaginal hysterectomy.

Dry vagina is more likely to occur months or years into postmenopause (except when it results from oophorectomy, which produces a sudden drop in estrogen levels). Dry vagina may be detected during regular medical examinations when insertion of the fingers or a speculum is found to be painful. More often, however, a woman notices that penetration by a penis is now uncomfortable.

Dyspareunia, or painful intercourse, continues to be viewed as almost solely a problem of postmenopausal women despite the fact that, according to at least one study, more than 30 percent of women in their thirties experience it occasionally or often. Doctors rarely inquire about painful intercourse when dealing with younger women, but it's a standard question put to women past fifty; this may add to an inflated estimate of the problem during postmenopause.

Healthy tissue in and around the vagina may be maintained by switching to natural fibers, which allow better air circulation. This means wearing cotton panties and pantyhose with cotton crotches or with the diamond-shaped gusset snipped out. Some women prefer to wear stockings with garters. Skirts are preferable to slacks, particularly if the slacks are tight-fitting. This may not be important for a younger woman, because the labia (lips) around the vagina tend to seal it; with age, the labia become less efficient. If you have a tendency to vaginitis, sitting in a hot tub or Jacuzzi where bacteria proliferate may create problems.

> My greatest problem is urinary leakage. Intercourse has become uncomfortable for me because of this. It is most distressing. The doctors and the specialist I have seen say there is nothing that can be done.

Many women notice the need to urinate more frequently, even though they are voiding smaller amounts (urge incontinence), or dribbling involuntarily when coughing, sneezing, or during orgasm (stress incontinence). Both conditions result from the thinning and shortening of tissue in the genitourinary tract and relaxation of the pelvic floor due to aging.

One can adapt to frequent urination, but the best way to prevent leakage is to do Kegel exercises regularly. These exercises, developed by Dr. Arnold Kegel, involve isolating the sphincter muscle (which controls urination) and strengthening it. If you faithfully practice tightening and loosening this muscle—an exercise that can be done anytime and anywhere—you may find that it alleviates not only incontinence problems, but also enhances the ability to respond sexually.

KEGEL EXERCISES

To locate your pubococcygeal (PC) muscle, simply stop your flow while urinating; it's the PC muscle that contracts to do this. Practice a few times to get the feeling of this muscle. Stop and start urinating at will. Try some stronger and weaker contractions until you can contract this muscle when not urinating. This will help you become familiar with this muscle. You can do your PC exercises anytime you wish; while waiting for a bus or walking down the street, or just after waking. Try them in fitness class when you are working on your abdominals—especially during the pelvic tilt. These two exercises go well together.

Three and Three
Contract your PC muscle for 3 full seconds and then release it for 3 seconds. Repeat 6 times, 3 times a day for a few days. Then repeat 12 times a day for a week.

One and One
Contract your PC muscle strongly for one second and release it for one second. Repeat 20 times, 3 times a day. Speed up the contractions so that you get a "fluttering" feeling here.

Ten and Five
Contract the PC muscle for 10 full seconds, working at holding the intensity of the contraction for the full period of time. Relax for 5 seconds. Repeat 5 times, 3 times a day.

Elevator
As you become more aware of your PC muscle, you will notice that you can feel the difference between your anal and vaginal muscle area. When you start to feel this difference, try the "elevator." Start with an anal contraction (bottom floor) and then move it along the PC muscle into the vaginal area and up to the "top floor." Repeat 6 times, 3 times a day.

Once you have improved your PC muscle tone and can do all of these exercises competently, try maintaining the strength and endurance of your PC muscle by doing your exercises once a day instead of three times. As with most exercise routines, it helps to set aside a specific time and place to ensure that you don't forget.

Source: *Fitness Leader,* September 1983

Nonprescription Remedies

Vaginal discharges should be monitored very carefully. Cutting down on dairy products, sugar, and artificial sweeteners may help chronic vaginal infections. Although a douche may give temporary relief, it is not a cure. Nonspecific vaginitis often recurs; based on a study of women prone to recurring vaginitis, regular consumption of nonpasteurized yogurt containing acidophilus lactobillus—8 oz. daily—was found to reduce such episodes by half.

Over-the-counter products are available (and heavily promoted) to relieve vaginitis, but if there is constant irritation, a change in color of discharge, or an unpleasant odor, make an appointment with your doctor to have it properly diagnosed and treated.

To prevent dry vagina, practice regular orgasm (which encourages natural lubrication) and Kegel exercises. If you do not have a regular partner, you might consciously decide to masturbate in order to keep your vagina healthy. If you do have a partner but find intercourse occasionally painful, this may be the time to explore other forms of sexual expression including oral/genital sex and mutual masturbation.

Many women find intercourse more comfortable with the help of saliva, a water-based lubricant (such as K-Y jelly or Lubafax), or a vitamin E suppository. These products are available at the drugstore and can be inserted into the vagina or smeared on the penis prior to penetration. Note that, despite all jokes to the contrary, petroleum-based lubricants such as Vaseline are not recommended, because they may damage fragile vaginal tissue. Astroglide and Replens are newer products that many women find helpful, despite the cost and, in the case of Replens, the environmentally wasteful overpackaging. Some women feel ashamed about having to use supplementary lubrication during sex, but many young couples depend on water-based lubricants for comfortable intercourse. Buying a tube of lubricant is not necessarily proclaiming middle-age inadequacy!

Preliminary evaluations of the new "woman's condom" or vaginal sheath suggest that this may also be useful in protecting the vagina from direct and painful friction during intercourse.

Because dryness of the vagina is partially due to a change in the chemical environment, some women have had success using natural yogurt internally to restore a healthy vaginal climate. Rosetta Reitz, in *Menopause: A Positive Approach*, recommends equal amounts of yogurt and a polyunsaturated oil both as a weekly regimen to keep the vaginal walls elastic, and also as a way of lubricating oneself prior to intercourse. Yogurt can be inserted into the vagina using the kind of applicator available with douches or foam spermicide, with a plastic tampon inserter, or with a turkey baster! Because of the consistency of this solution, it is better to be horizontal and to remain horizontal for some time after insertion. And you may want to place a towel under you to protect the bedclothes—or the bearskin rug, depending on your mood!

The tissues outside the vagina, sometimes the whole area around the crotch, may become dry and itchy. If you are already wearing cotton next to the skin, itchiness can often be relieved using "hygienic wipes"—small pads of cotton that are impregnated with witch hazel and glycerin. You can find hygienic wipes at the drugstore, often close to products for hemorrhoid relief. Other products that help to soothe prickly itch are pure shortening and cornstarch. If the itchiness is serious and is felt inside the vagina, you may have developed some kind of dermatitis or perhaps contracted an infection, so consult a dermatologist. As the tissues thin out, many women become more vulnerable to infections that are not necessarily sexually transmitted.

If you find that you are prone to recurrent bouts of cystitis (bladder infections that produce a burning sensation when urinating), make a habit of drinking large quantities of water. Drinking cranberry or blueberry juice on a regular basis also helps to combat the bacteria responsible for such infections. Avoid using a diaphragm, because this has been associated with increased risk of cystitis. If possible, avoid progesterone (either alone or in conjunction with estrogen) because this may aggravate bladder trouble.

Incontinence is no longer regarded as a normal corollary of growing older (or many pregnancies). In addition to practicing Kegel exercises, it is possible to retrain the bladder by timing visits to the toilet; going every hour, then every 90 minutes, then every 120 minutes, until it is possible to stay comfortable and dry for three-hour stretches. Some urologists also advocate the use of vaginal cones, which are available in graduated sizes and are held inside the vagina for stipulated periods of time in order to strengthen the pelvic muscles. Others recommend collagen injections to strengthen the sphincter muscle and ensure continence. No matter what the problem, a sympathetic urologist should be helpful in finding a solution.

Prescription Remedies

Estrogen cream is commonly prescribed for dry vagina. It is recommended that ten days of oral estrogen precede use of the cream, but this guideline is not universally followed. It is not advisable to take two forms of estrogen, so if you are taking tablets, using the patch, or have had an injection, report this to your doctor. Estrogen cream comes with its own applicator calibrated in grams for insertion into the vagina. The recommended dosage on the package is 2 to 4 grams daily, on a cycle of three weeks on and one week off. This is often more than most women need.

The most popular estrogen cream is Premarin, which contains .625 mg of conjugated estrogen *per gram*. Because estrogen cream is absorbed into the system—with effects on the whole body, not just on the problem area—use of 2 to 4 grams of cream daily is potentially equivalent to a daily dose, in oral tablets, of from 1.25 to 2.5 mg, or 2 to 4 times the normal amount. (The amount absorbed is partly dependent on the fragility of the tissue.) Most women find that a fraction of this amount will serve to restore the vagina, although it may take three weeks to reverse the situation. Once the vagina is comfortable again, you can experiment with less frequent use—perhaps two weeks on and two weeks off or, after time, one week of regular use of the cream every month.

The applicator supplied tends to deposit the cream deep into the vagina, but it should also be smeared just inside the opening of the vagina, which is the area that is usually most painful. Estrogen cream, unlike water-based lubricants, is a medication and should *not* be used just prior to intercourse since it will be absorbed by your partner as well. If you have an intact uterus and use estrogen vaginal cream over a period of months, a course of synthetic progesterone may be advisable every three to six months to make sure that excess endometrial cells are sloughed off.

Antibiotics are often prescribed for cystitis and will usually solve the problem. If the problem recurs and antibiotics seem ineffective, however, you may be dealing with a case of interstitial cystitis, which requires a different approach. Information about this is available from the Interstitial Cystitis Association (see the end of this chapter). Treatment for vaginitis will depend on the diagnosis but will often involve the woman and her partner.

For chronic vulvar itch (or vestibulitis—inflammation of the outer part of the vagina), a dermatologist may prescribe a cortisone cream. Although this often solves the problem, cortisone cream may occasionally contribute to *added* thinning of the tissue and merely compound the problem. If you do use cortisone cream, use it sparingly and monitor yourself. (Use a hand mirror to examine the color and texture of the tissue.)

Irregularity of periods, hot flashes and night sweats, and genito-urinary distress are legitimate concerns that you may wish to discuss with your doctor. You deserve a sympathetic and supportive hearing and, because these complaints are commonly associated with menopause, you will probably receive some counsel about the advantages and disadvantages of medication.

(Osteoporosis is often a *concern* at menopause but it is not, strictly speaking, a menopausal ailment. It starts well before the menopause years and becomes a problem for most women after menopause is past. It is discussed in chapter 6.)

Despite the recent publicity given to menopause, there are many other menopausal complaints that are rarely discussed. This may be because these ailments are often not relieved by ET or CHT. If it's true that menopausal ailments are caused by an estrogen deficiency, then supplementary estrogen should be the perfect remedy for every menopausal complaint. Unfortunately, this is not the case.

Joint Pain

If you experience joint pain, you should check with a doctor. If tests for arthritis are negative, however, chances are that the pain is associated with menopause and is a temporary nuisance. Many women have found that extra vitamin B_6 (1.5–2.0 mg daily), or combinations of vitamin C and cod liver oil (vitamin D), relieve the ache. Your doctor may suggest a cortisone shot (which masks the pain without relieving the cause), or you may consult a physiotherapist about appropriate exercises to ease the stiffness and/or pain. However, for all those women (including myself) who have been diagnosed with frozen shoulder or tennis elbow or housemaid's knee or carpal tunnel syndrome or heel spurs or sore thumbs, or any other affliction that is more annoying than incapacitating, it may be advisable to wait it out. It may just go away.

Migraine

Migraine headaches have been a bane of mine for years, but they have had no regularity. Mine fall into the "common" category. Sometimes I feel they are caused by food allergies, cosmetics, smoke, and stress. I usually wake up in the morning with a migraine, don't have any warning symptoms, and the bad ones last three days, with nausea, vomiting (which usually provides relief), a peculiar metallic taste in my mouth, and a feeling of general malaise.

Countless experiments have been conducted to alleviate migraine with hormonal preparations—estrogens, progesterones, combinations of these and other hormones. But because so many young women suffer their first migraine after starting on the pill, and because the hormonal status responsible is not yet understood, migraine sufferers are generally discouraged from taking any form of supplementary hormones. Since the blood vessels in the head are dilated during migraine, there is concern that hormone use might promote blood clot formation; these clots might loosen, be carried into the brain, and cause a stroke.

Migraines can be triggered by such things as loss of sleep, oversleep, fasting (low blood sugar), falling barometric pressure, glaring sunshine, and flickering fluorescent or strobe lights. Many migraine sufferers (the correct term is *migraineurs*) cannot adequately process foods containing certain types of amines, although the headache may not start for hours after eating the foods responsible. Some of the most common culprits are aged cheese (cheddar), chocolate, vinegar, sour cream, yogurt, yeast products, nuts, onions, citrus fruits, bananas, pork, caffeine-rich beverages, cured cold meats, and alcohol. This reaction to food is not an allergy in the common sense of the term; the amine-containing substance can only rarely be isolated using standard allergy tests.

More mysterious than the migraine headache is the *migraine equivalent,* a disturbance that appears to be generated in the same way as the headache but without the ache. Migraine equivalents may be merely the aura (or prodrome) of the headache—spots in front of the eyes, disturbed vision, dizzy spells—or may manifest themselves in effects on one side of the body—a pain down one side, a glowing red ear, a throbbing or dull ache in the abdomen. The variations are many but these weird experiences seem to become more common as menopause approaches. It may take determination and persistence to find a well-informed neurologist who can offer support and understanding.

Other migraineurs may have yeast infections (systemic candida albicans, an overgrowth of a normal flora found in the body) or temporomandibular jaw (TMJ) syndrome (faulty articulation of the hinged joint of the jawbone; a condition that may cause, in addition to headache, dizziness or ringing in the ears). It is suspected that tendency to migraine may also result from a major trauma in childhood, such as physical or sexual abuse.

As soon as a migraine starts, the most effective therapy is to lie down in a quiet, darkened room. Other preventive measures are splashing the face with cold water, or stepping into a steamy, hot shower (to dilate the blood vessels in the head) and then gradually switching to cold water (to contract the blood vessels). Not an inviting prospect!

Many migraineurs have learned to control their headaches with variations of biofeedback, relaxation therapy, and visualization. Biofeedback is usually taught at a headache or pain clinic and frequently includes exercises in progressive relaxation. One form of biofeedback teaches the person to raise the temperature of the hands using visual imagery (i.e., imagining one's hands in the sun, or dipped in a basin of warm water). As the hands warm up, the headache starts to go away. Another visualizing technique is to concentrate on the image of a headache as contained in a glaring light bulb. Then, by using the full power of imagination, the light bulb is gradually dimmed. All such techniques require supervised practice initially, but once mastered, frequently provide an effective way to control migraine and, at the same time, to break the reliance on drugs.

Today, more credence is given to the very real pain experienced by many migraine sufferers. If you have exhausted other possibilities and are unwilling to rely on drugs for relief, it might be worthwhile to inquire about a pain clinic at your nearest large hospital.

Nonprescription Remedies

Over-the-counter preparations—acetaminophen (Panadol, Tylenol), or aspirin may be useful if taken immediately at onset and/or for mild migraines. Preparations containing codeine are not recommended because they are addictive and may cause nausea or vomiting. In Britain, research at the University of Nottingham has demonstrated that the herb feverfew (chrysanthemum parthenium) has the ability to ward off or reduce the severity of a migraine. Because feverfew is not available in standardized doses, use of this herbal remedy requires a bit of experimentation.

Prescription Remedies

The standard prescription drug is ibuprofen (Advil, Motrin, etc.)—some brands of which may be purchased over the counter. In about 50 percent of cases, ergotamine tartrate (Ergomar, Ergostat, etc.), taken immediately at onset, wards off or shortens the migraine. Ergotamine is available in tablet form, in an inhaler, as a suppository or by injection. Variations are ergot-and-caffeine (Cafergot), ergot-caffeine-belladonna-and-phenobarbital (Cafergot PB), and belladonna-ergot-and-phenobarbital (Bellergal and Bellergal Spacetabs). Frequent use of any ergot preparation is dangerous. Migraineurs who use ergot must remain under medical supervision to prevent overuse and rebound headaches, which may be even worse.

A new and promising prescription drug is succinate of sumitriptan, marketed as Imitrex (by Glaxo), which is now available in auto-injectors. It is very expensive, but one self-administered injection may be enough to halt a migraine in its tracks. There is some concern about adverse effects (chest pains, breathlessness) and these will have to be investigated before Imitrex is fully accepted.

Migraines that occur more often than two or three times a month may be treated with preventive drugs. Beta-blockers are often prescribed, but beware of side effects. Propranolol (Inderal), for instance, often causes restless sleep with frequent awakenings. Calcium blockers, anti-inflammatories and antidepressants may also be employed in an effort to prevent migraines. In fact, the wide range of drugs used in an attempt to halt migraines is an indication of the enormous puzzle that migraine poses. Any of these medications has potential side effects. None should be taken for more than a few months.

Burning Mouth Syndrome

Four years ago, in the middle of the afternoon, my mouth caught fire. And it remained that way for three years! For a few hours, I put it down to something I ate. After a few days, I became suspicious that it might be something more serious. After a few weeks, I saw my doctor. Over the months since, I have seen many doctors—a family physician, dermatologist, allergist, and dentist. No one could diagnose the problem. To relieve it, I tried sucking on Popsicles, ice cubes, mints, or chewing gum—anything wet or cold. A year later, I heard on the news that a mysterious disease had doctors baffled.

Patients were complaining of a burning mouth and tongue. It was now recognized as a genuine disorder. I felt vindicated! The symptoms persisted for another year, but I took comfort in the fact that I was not alone.

Although we know that dry mouth can result from too much caffeine or too many antihistamines, burning mouth syndrome is harder to treat. Sucking on ice cubes or peppermint lozenges, and drinking cold water are the usual responses to this syndrome, but the only lasting relief has been found by massaging the gums. Because it is assumed that this condition is related to changes inside the vagina (the tissue involved is similar), studies have been done using vitamin E oil or estrogen cream as a "massage agent." Both appear to be equally effective; it is massage that seems to make the difference. The only good news about burning mouth syndrome is that it goes away after a while and that it is now being taken more seriously by the medical and dental professions, with research projects underway into causes and possible remedies.

Indigestion, Flatulence, Bloat

During middle-age, many persons (both men and women) develop lactose intolerance, and find milk and milk products (with the exception of yogurt) difficult to digest. For some, garlic, green pepper, or cucumber may suddenly create problems. Foods high in fat often cause heartburn. All of this is very common and undoubtedly due more to aging—and to changes in the amount and efficacy of gastric acid—than to menopause. However, it often shows up for the first time during the menopausal years. Perhaps you should keep a log of the foods you eat so that you can do some detective work.

If you notice excess gas after drinking milk or eating cheese, you may want to buy a lactase enzyme. These products are sold in drugstores and health food stores, in liquid or tablet form. When added to milk, which must then sit for a few hours, it predigests the lactose. You can then have the benefit of the calcium in the milk without the problem of indigestion. Yogurt, although technically a milk product, is often easier to digest than milk or cheese and may help the body to digest other foods high in lactose.

In addition, foods high in potassium—such as bananas, apricots, tomato, or orange juice—may relieve excess gas, and may also help to reduce the risk of stroke! Papaya tablets or activated charcoal (both available at health food stores) also prevent that terrible gassy feeling.

> Gas problems have been an embarrassment for several
> years. I initially put the blame on irregular hours,
> eating habits, diet, what have you. I tried eliminating
> certain foods and adding others. Meat seemed to be hard
> to digest so I tried some papaya tablets. When the papaya
> helped somewhat, I got a stronger version. It solved
> my problem with flatulence completely.

Bloat is somewhat of a mystery. It may very well occur as a result of eating some of the foods mentioned, but it also seems to happen for no reason at all. I vividly remember surreptitiously unzipping my jeans at the dinner table one evening and then finding, to my consternation, that I could not zip them up again! My waist size had suddenly increased by two to three inches, although it was back to normal the next morning. Keep track of what you eat, but remember that bloat is fairly common and that these episodes disappear with time.

Sleep Problems

As we age, we tend to need less and less sleep but, whereas men's need for sleep seems to diminish gradually, many women suddenly find themselves wide awake in the middle of the night, or regularly waking with the first light of dawn. Room-darkening shades or blindfolds are often effective. A glass of warm milk before bed is an effective remedy, because warm milk releases tryptophan, an amino acid that is an effective and mild sleep-inducer. Antihistamines prepared to relieve motion sickness (dimenhydrinate or Gravol) or cold symptoms (Dristan, Contac-C, Chlor-Trimeton) may also induce drowsiness.

Regular exercise improves the quality of sleep. Many women find that a walk after dinner will help them to fall asleep more easily. Practitioners of yoga can teach their bodies to relax, since deep breathing invites sleep. Some women find progressive relaxation helpful. Audiotapes that give instructions in this technique are available from sleep clinics, clinical psychologists, or through advertisements in magazines dealing with health and well-being.

Although sleep apnea is more common among men, if you awaken frequently gasping for breath, or if you begin to snore very loudly, you may want to be checked at a Sleep Lab (or clinic) in your local hospital. Or you may find an experimental psychologist interested in this problem; it may be worth calling the Psychology Department of your local university.

Routine sleeplessness is a temporary aggravation of menopause. It helps to realize just how much can be accomplished on very little sleep. I hear from women who bake, or read, or write letters, or watch old movies for an hour or two in the middle of the night. And yet they put in a full day's work every day! The stamina of the midlife woman is admirable.

Prescription Remedies

If sleeplessness due to hot flashes or night sweats leads to intolerable fatigue, a short course of estrogen may help. ET may contribute to more restful sleep by allowing one to fall asleep more quickly (reducing "sleep latency") and adding to the ratio of dream sleep. The amount of dream sleep is one criterion for the quality of sleep, sleep that leaves you feeling refreshed. In fact, sleepers who are deprived of dream sleep exhibit abnormally high levels of anxiety.

Sleeping pills, conversely, *reduce* the amount of dream sleep. If you cannot or will not take estrogen and depression is *not* a problem, you may want to ask your doctor to prescribe a mild tranquilizer. Tranquilizers are not as soporific as sleeping pills and are less likely to cause a "drugged" feeling the next morning. But remember, tranquilizers are depressants and can be addictive, so don't use them unless you know that it will be a "sometime" thing—once every ten days or two weeks. If you know that you have addictive tendencies, don't use them. If you find you are using them more often, flush them away.

Weight Gain

Even when one is aware of the benefits to bones and the alleviation of hot flashes, it is hard to accept living with a weight gain of ten to fifteen pounds. If weight soars beyond this extra cushion of fat—to 20 percent of ideal weight, the threshold of obesity—one is inviting a host of medical problems. The only solution to permanent weight loss is a long period of sensible eating and a loss of no more than two pounds a week. Prolonged diets have the advantage of inducing improved eating habits, including a sharp cutback in alcoholic beverages. Weight gain is discussed more fully in Chapter 8.

Other Complaints

Skin and Hair

Dry hair and dry skin are often improved by regular exercise, which seems to lubricate the system generally. Dry skin benefits from products that use a base of petrolatum or lanolin. It is not necessary to buy expensive products. The "crawling skin" sensation can be relieved by ET, but I have heard from a number of women who have used homeopathic remedies successfully for this complaint.

Hair may appear to thin out as the texture changes to gray. And hair may also thin either as a result of excess estrogen in the system, or as a result of the influence of androgens. Some women find that starting estrogen supplements will halt hair loss, whereas others find that stopping estrogen (or losing a substantial amount of weight) achieves the same effect.

If you are convinced that you are losing an inordinate amount of hair, you might want to consult a specialist who may prescribe spironolactone, an antiandrogen that is often used to treat women with excess body hair but which, paradoxically, often helps to restore frontal hair loss on the head. Because spironolactone has powerful and often unpleasant side effects, milder remedies—such as a herbal rinse made of stinging nettles—may be more appealing. Minoxidil (Rogaine) is being strongly promoted to relieve hair loss but it's expensive, takes about eight months of daily application to determine its effectiveness, works for only 30 to 40 percent of those who try it, and must be used for life. Side effects include itching and prickling, headaches, dizzy spells or lightheadedness, and irregular heartbeat. It is also too early to know about possible long-term effects.

Allergies and Sensitivities

Despite the fact that any other period of hormonal fluctuation—such as puberty, pregnancy, and childbirth—is known to be a time of onset of, and sometimes remission from, allergies and sensitivities, there is no official evidence that this also holds true for menopause. However, the anecdotal evidence—hundreds of letters that I have received—convince me that this is a fairly common occurrence.

Be alert to newly developed sensitivities. I have found that my eyes run when the wind is cold—a form of rhinitis (inflammation of the nose) that may have something to do with urban pollution, but which certainly started during menopause. Other women report that they now have a bad reaction to cigarette smoke. Some women have found that certain foods—wheat, for instance—add to a sense of fatigue.

> My problem is one I've never heard anyone else mention—
> bruises. They are large or small and resemble the type
> of surface bruise incurred when you bump yourself.
> However, I'm sure I haven't bumped myself and they
> seem to get worse when my flashes are more frequent.

If you experience one of the more unusual ailments—tachycardia (rapid heartbeat), mysterious bruises, attacks of dizziness, "rubber legs,"—keep track of when and where you experience it. Tachycardia may be due to mitral valve prolapse (to be checked out with a cardiologist) but, if no cause can be found for it, relief may sometimes be found by adding magnesium to the diet. Dizziness may be a migraine equivalent. In all cases of suspected menopausal ailments, try to figure out if something happened in the past that might account for it. Have you had any similar experiences before? What have you done to try to make yourself feel better? Your complaint may or may not be taken seriously, but a conscientious doctor will order tests to rule out conditions that might cause the same or similar complaints. You may have to do without the firm professional assurance that it is related to menopause, but you may be relieved to find that you are generally healthy.

One of the most common remedies offered to menopausal women is the tranquilizer, a drug that is both addictive and a depressant. With the sole exception of sleeplessness, which may be relieved by the infrequent use of a mild tranquilizer, none of the physical ailments discussed in this chapter call for a prescription for alprazolam (Xanax), lorazepam (Ativan), or diazepam (Valium). Doctors may offer a prescription not because they know it will alleviate a particular complaint, but because they know that patients *expect* to leave with a prescription. It is the concluding ritual of the appointment and a way of validating the patient's complaint. If your doctor can only suggest tranquilizers, you may want to find another physician, or to consult with another kind of health practitioner.

REFERENCES AND RESOURCES

Albers, M. M. "Osteoporosis: A health issue for women," *Health Care for Women Internatl.*, 11:11–19:1990.

Asthma and Allergy Foundation, 1717 Massachusetts Ave., Suite 305, Washington, DC 20036. (Patient Information Line, 800–7–ASTHMA.)

Burgio, K. L., K. L. Pearce, and A. J. Lucco. *Staying Dry: A Practical Guide to Bladder Control.* Baltimore: Johns Hopkins University Press, 1990.

Fantl, J. A., J. F. Wyman, R. L. Anderson et al. "Postmenopausal urinary incontinence: Comparison between non-estrogen-supplemented and estrogen-supplemented women," *Obs. & Gyn.*, 71(6) June 1988.

Gannon, L. "The potential role of exercise in the alleviation of menstrual disorders and menopause symptoms: A theoretical synthesis of recent research." *Women & Health*, 14(2):105–127:1988.

Gillespie, L. *You Don't Have to Live with Cystitis.* NY: Rawson Associates, 1987.

Hartmann, E. *The Sleep Book: Understanding and Preventing Sleep Problems in People over 50.* Glenview, IL: Scott Foresman, 1987.

Henig, R. M. *The Myth of Senility: The Truth about the Brain and Aging (rev. ed.).* Glenview, IL: Scott Foresman, 1985.

HIP (Help for Incontinent People) Report, quarterly newsletter available from HIP Inc., Box 544, Union, SC 29379. (Resource guide and other publications also available.)

ICA Update, quarterly newsletter available from the Interstitial Cystitis Association, P.O. Box 1553, Madison Sq. Station, New York, NY 10159.

The Informer, quarterly newsletter on incontinence available from The Simon Foundation, P.O. Box 815, Wilmette, IL 60091 (800-23-SIMON).

National Headache Foundation Newsletter, quarterly newsletter of the National Headache Foundation, 5252 North Western Ave., Chicago, IL 60625 (800-843-2256; 800-523-8858 in IL).

Reitz, R. *Menopause: A Positive Approach.* NY: Penguin, 1979.

Seaman, B. and G. Seaman. *Women and the Crisis in Sex Hormones.* NY: Rawson Associates, 1977.

Sherwin, B. B. "Estrogen and/or androgen replacement therapy and cognitive functioning in surgical menopausal women," *Psychoneuroendocrinology, 13:*345–357, 1988.

Slick, R. G. *Herbs for Menopause.* East Barre, VT: Sage (no date).

Smith. W. *Overcoming Cystitis: A Practical Self-help Guide for Women.* NY: Bantam Books, 1986.

"Test points out high-risk postmenopausal women," and "Calcium supplements: Role re-assessed," in: Meeting highlights from the International Symposium on Osteoporosis, Aalborg, Denmark: *Geriatrics, 43*(5);90:May 1988.

Urinary Incontinence in Adults, free from Agency for Health Care Policy and Research, Publications Clearinghouse, P.O. Box 8547, Silver Spring, MD 20907.

Voda, A. M. *Menopause Me & You: A Personal Handbook for Women.* College of Nursing, University of Utah, 25 S. Medical Drive, Salt Lake City, UT 84112.

Walz, T. H. and N. S. Blum. *Sexual Health in Later Life.* Lexington, MA: D.C. Health, 1987.

4

Psychological and Sexual Effects

This chapter deals with psychological and sexual effects of menopause separately from other ailments, not because they are any less important than physical ailments, but because they require a different approach. Many women who freely admit to hot flashes turn suddenly shy when talking about panic attacks or loss of sexual desire. The causes of each of these may be similar—a temporary biochemical disturbance—but less is known about the psychology and sexuality of menopause. Because the precise hormonal interactions are so poorly understood, no standard diagnosis or treatment has been formulated.

Physicians are thus often ill-equipped to conduct discussions of mood swings, anxiety, panic attacks, and depression. When they refer their patients to a psychologist or psychiatrist, the patient feels that her problem is being redefined as emotional or mental, when *she* believes that it is due to stress on the *body*.

In the same way, sexual problems involve not only the physical responses of the woman but the complex attitudes and feelings of the woman and her partner as well. If physicians are ill-equipped to handle psychological complaints, they are even more uncomfortable with sexual questions. It helps to know that, although some psychological and sexual effects require medical expertise, others may be solved through increased self-knowledge or better communication, and that both of these can often be facilitated by a qualified therapist.

Psychological Problems

Memory Lapses

Menopausal forgetfulness is not something that most doctors care to discuss, nor do most women wish to bring it up. Many of us joke, somewhat uneasily, about the onset of Alzheimer's disease, although most Alzheimer victims apparently aren't aware of their failing memories. However, *we* feel the lack and, for many women, part of the frustration is having this faltering memory brought to their attention. Women have traditionally remembered the birthdays, the items needed at the store, the names of casual acquaintances. Now we feel we are letting others down. Again, a sense of loss.

Of all the psychological effects of menopause, forgetfulness is probably the most common. We are told that this is due to age, that we have too much on our minds, that it is due to stress, and that men have it, too. We are also directed to articles that teach us how to remember—mnemonic exercises to help us remember names or items on a list.

Last year, I could go to the supermarket and remember ten items without a list. This year, I walk upstairs to get *one* thing and forget why I went upstairs. Last year, I knew the first names of all the wives of my husband's club members whom I see once every six months; this year, I remembered the names of two. Yesterday, I put the bread in the freezer and the ice cubes in the breadbox. Today, I'm buying another notebook to keep yet more lists.

Some nutritionists believe that memory lapses are partly due to a deficiency of a particular kind of lecithin (a phospholipid found in eggs and seeds); other experts say that the body manufactures all the lecithin we need. Preliminary studies tell us that removal of the ovaries may result in perceptible differences in the ability to concentrate and to retain information. Such differences are not so noticeable among naturally menopausal women. And the deficits that *do* exist are not significant. Even at its worst, menopausal forgetfulness is no worse and no different than would be considered within the range of normal in any other context, or with any other group. Perhaps menopause is the time for women to abandon their self-imposed role of "memory bank" for the boss, husband, and children. The ability to concentrate, together with attention span and memory, appears to improve after the worst of menopause. Perhaps, unlike male memory, female memory takes a sudden nosedive at menopause and then levels off again.

Anxiety

Many women find that the onset of menopause makes them more anxious. They become fraught with worry over chores that were once routine. A teacher is suddenly self-conscious in front of her class; an executive is filled with self-doubt prior to a routine presentation to a client; a hostess worries herself sick about a run-of-the-mill dinner party. Such women are victims of "free-floating anxiety" that afflicts many women as they enter menopause. The anxiety does not seem linked to any particular event; it is simply there. What was once considered new and fun becomes worrisome and even frightening. Many women force themselves to take on new challenges, and at the same time feel great empathy for women who find that routine chores are almost more than they can handle. Like many other facets of menopause, these flurries of anxiety—particularly when faced with the new and untried—are likely to be temporary. It may be some comfort to think about the countless menopausal women lying in bed at night, self-consciously reviewing their stupidities of that day—an activity they had intended to give up at age fifteen!

One problem with anxiety is that it is so relative. Some women are anxious all the time and, although probably thought of as highstrung, appear to function adequately if not serenely. Anxiety is a form of neuroticism, and the border line between normal neuroticism (we're all neurotic about something) and anxiety depends on the degree and the duration. Anxiety becomes debilitating when it seriously hampers one's regular activities over a long period of time. Persons who make radical changes to established routine in order to avoid stressful situations, and who maintain this avoidance behavior for months, are exceeding ordinary anxiety. If the disorder persists, it may become phobic, and professional help should be sought; this occurs only rarely.

For most of us, it is comforting to know that the sense of anxiety is shared, that many other women are feeling the same way and that, like many of our physical woes, it will go away in time. Meanwhile, perhaps we should order our nearest and dearest to refrain from expressions like, "Don't worry," "Just relax," or (the one I hate), "Lighten up, will you?" We will stop worrying and start relaxing when we are no longer feeling so anxious. And we will let the Pollyannas around us know when this happens!

Irritability

Irritability is even more visible than anxiety. We get angry about things that never bothered us before. We shake with rage over a trifling matter. The puzzlement we feel about our own behavior is often reinforced by puzzled looks on the faces of close friends, coworkers, or family members. It is worth considering whether irritability is more of a problem for you (the woman) or for those close to you. Many women are more concerned about the effect they have on others than they are about themselves. This leads to a situation where a woman seeks help or accepts medication for the benefit of those who tell her that she is not "herself." Unwilling to ask others to adjust to this newly-willful person, the woman may accept some sort of chemical help (usually a tranquilizer) to restore her amiability.

While it is true that menopausal women can be unusually bitchy, they can also be unusually assertive, creative, and self-protective. It is *not* that a particular incident now irritates when it never irritated before. It's just that they are not willing to put up with that particular irritant one more time. It may be that they're not feeling well (and therefore it irritates more); it may be something that has always been vexing and it is now time to speak out about it. Because menopause makes us sharply conscious of aging, we are more aware of the life we have left to live, and often super-conscious of the annoying traits and behaviors of those around us. We may never have mentioned it before, but the prospect of living with it (whatever "it" is) any longer may be intolerable.

Looked at in another way, many women come into their own at menopause. They have put the needs of others first for many years. Menopause may be the trigger that makes women demand their fair share for the first time. Sometimes this newfound assertiveness is channeled into a new enterprise, whether hobby or work. The sense of impatience, of too much to do and not enough time in which to do it, persuades women to return to school, to take up new challenges, to give up chores and responsibilities that have chafed or bored. There are many positive aspects to this "irritability."

In order to survive, I needed blocks of unfractured time
and private space. Our children usually have rooms
of their own; our parents have living space of their
own. We, mothers and wives, may lay partial claim to
a "master bedroom" (and hear what I am saying because
we use words without thinking). A woman I spoke
to not long ago said that what she wants is to find
a dark closet somewhere and get some peace. I suggested
a more daring approach—her own room in the house!
And not a sewing room or a corner of the living-room
either!

When I found myself sighing and sometimes crying
in the bathroom (often after having waited to get in),
I knew I was in deep trouble.

The standard "remedy" for anxiety and irritability is a
tranquilizer. If you accept a prescription, be sure that you do
so for your *own* benefit, not merely to pacify those around
you. Be aware also that it is potentially addictive and a depressant. If you are already feeling depressed, as well as
anxious and irritable (a common situation), the tranquilizer
will make you feel *more* depressed.

Panic Attacks

After turning fifty, I suddenly found myself drenched
in perspiration while out shopping, experiencing some
very nasty dizzy spells and feelings of unreality, and
I began to dread the daily trips to the supermarket.
After a while, I began dropping my purchases and
making a beeline for the nearest exit and home; the
worst thing I could have done, of course, as counseling
has since taught me! But try telling that to a person
having a bad panic attack. They wouldn't stay around
long enough to listen to you, let alone heed your good
advice!

Frankly, I am convinced that the chemical and hormonal imbalance that menopause brings about *does* play a very large part in upsetting our equilibrium. Some of us manage to muddle through somehow without falling apart at the seams. Others become so afraid that they become housebound.

Panic attacks, a more focused form of anxiety—and, fortunately, relatively rare—involve the body as well as the mind. During a panic attack, adrenaline rushes into the bloodstream, the heart pounds, the palms of the hands sweat, and breathing becomes quick and shallow. Although the attack is undoubtedly caused by some sudden change in brain chemistry, the mind seems to seize on some*one* or some*thing* as a cause. Suddenly, out of nowhere, we imagine a terrible accident about to happen to a loved one, or something unspeakably embarrassing that we are about to do, such as faint, or fall over. It is only after the panic abates that we realize that the pounding heart and quick breathing came *first*, that the situation itself did not *cause* the panic attack.

Many menopausal women deal with panic attacks by breathing slowly and deeply, and by counting, singing, whistling, or reciting nursery rhymes (anything that drives away negative thoughts). Some women carry a small brown paper bag to breathe into, which often wards off hyperventilation—abnormally quick, shallow breathing. If the panic attacks are very severe or the recurrence is restricting activity in any way, it is time to get help. A good psychotherapist can provide the tools to enable you to get past this kind of block.

It would be helpful to have an explanation for these bizarre menopausal effects but, so far, no one has been able to trace the effects of brain chemistry on specific behaviors such as these. Menopause, by itself, may be a source of stress for the body, and this stress often adds to existing stress—stress imposed by the burden of commitments in the roles of wife, daughter, mother, housekeeper, worker, friend. In other words, it is probably not menopause *itself* that induces anxiety (or irritability, or panic attacks) but rather the extra, added stress of menopause that is unbearable.

> I have come to the conclusion that the mind tries to give a name or substance to its fears when attempting to deal with free-floating anxiety, and that just about anything will do. I am now fifty-six and panic far more easily than I ever did before middle age and the onset of "the change." To be honest, in the past few years, I find myself panicking over so many stupid little things that, in earlier years, I would have never given a second thought to.
>
> I also experience spells of great sadness at times and weep for no good reason. Sometimes there just seems to be an awful feeling of doom, as if something dreadful were about to happen. Just as quickly as these feelings come, they disappear.

Depression

Of all the psychological effects of menopause, the most dreaded is undoubtedly depression. Despite the fact that menopausal women are *less* likely to suffer from clinically diagnosed depression than are much younger women (particularly mothers of young children), depression continues to be a bugaboo. Not only are women frightened about being depressed but they're ashamed to admit that they *are* depressed. Somehow, this condition doesn't seem fitting for a "mature" woman in her forties or fifties. There is also the stigma of depression: depressed women have traditionally been treated as if they were personally responsible. They "didn't have enough to do" or "thought about themselves too much." Although these destructive attitudes linger on (it's called "blaming the victim") more and more we see that *some* women, for no known reason, *do* get depressed at menopause. This is much more likely to happen if the menopause is surgically induced, or if the woman has experienced a depression at some other stage in her life, but it also happens to women who believe they have absolutely no reason to feel depressed. Menopause affects brain chemistry, depression results from a temporary imbalance in brain chemistry, and depression is self-limiting. In other words, a depression will go away whether you seek help or not. For most of us, the biggest struggle is to acknowledge depression—either in oneself or in a friend.

Menopausal depressions almost never involve *bipolar depression*, a depression followed by a period of manic activity and energy, widely recognized as a genuine mental illness. It is rather a depression characterized by fatigue and an absence of a sense of purpose or of worth. According to the *Diagnostic & Statistical Manual of Mental Disorders*, 3rd edition Revised:

... the essential feature of a major depressive episode is either depressed mood or loss of interest or pleasure in all, or almost all, activities, and associated symptoms, for a period of at least two weeks. The symptoms represent a change from previous functioning and are relatively persistent, that is, they occur for most of the day, nearly every day, during at least a two-week period. The associated symptoms include appetite disturbance, change in weight, sleep disturbance, psychomotor agitation or retardation, decreased energy, feelings of worthlessness or excessive and inappropriate guilt, difficulty thinking or concentrating, and recurrent thoughts of death, or suicidal ideation or attempts.

Menopausal depression has been found to be abnormally high among women who have had hysterectomies and oophorectomies (occurring in from 55 to 75 percent of cases and peaking two years after the operation). However, depressed women are also more likely to *report* severe menopausal symptoms (to a clinic, or to their doctors), which may be why

depression is so often linked with menopause. It is often hard
to know which came first, the depression or the menopause.

> I am forty-seven and was not going through menopause
> until a hysterectomy completely devastated me a year
> ago. I knew nothing of menopause—had had no hot
> flashes nor depression. Now I can really relate to other
> women who are suffering these symptoms. I have had
> a terrible year. I find the depression worse than
> anything else. I wake up each morning with a silent
> prayer, "Please, God, let me have one good day so I can
> bear the rest." The odd good days keep me going. I have
> wonderful friends and a husband who is loving and
> caring. If it were not for his tender understanding,
> I would never get through.

There is no real agreement about the cause of depression,
but there are two main theories. The first is that depression
results from a reaction to the biological or social facts of being a woman. Women suffer from depression in numbers estimated to be from two to six times higher than the rate for
men. Depression may be "rage turned inward": women may
experience depression because they do not act out their anger in the same way that men do. Instead of venting resentment or hostility in verbal or physical ways, women
transform it into guilt, anxiety, or depression. The old term
for menopausal depression, *"involutional melancholia,"*
means an inward-turning sadness.

The depressed menopausal woman may be mourning—
mourning the loss of reproductive ability, mourning the babies she never had, mourning the opportunities missed,
mourning her loss of attractiveness. Or she may feel depressed because she has lost the socially valued role of
mother (which often coincides with menopause) and must
now confront the prospect of old age. There is a mourning,
but this is not so much a mourning of reproductive ability as
a mourning for the social role that had defined that woman's

place in her world. In her book, *Women and Madness*, Phyllis Chesler says, "Women are in a continual state of mourning—for what they never had, or had too briefly—and for what they can't have."

These explanations for midlife depression are all rooted in circumstances particular to the female. When we look at woman's role in this society, at the shockingly high rates of sexual and spousal abuse directed at females, we can understand how valid are women's deep-seated resentments, which may show themselves as depression.

There is also a biochemical basis for some kinds of depression. *Postpartum depression* (the kind of depression that follows childbirth, whether a temporary "blues" or a more long-standing condition) is assumed to be caused by an imbalance in hormones affecting brain chemistry (or brain chemistry that affects hormones). A woman who has just given birth moves into a high-risk category for depression as does the woman who has had a hysterectomy, whether or not the ovaries are left. No equivalent surgery (appendectomy, gallbladder surgery, etc.) produces the risk of depression that follows the trauma (natural or induced) to the female reproductive organs. Logically then, menopause *may* (not *will*) induce depression in a minority of women as a result of some kind of biochemical effect. In real life, of course, it is often difficult to distinguish between a depression that is biochemically caused and one that is triggered by social experience, present or past.

Some women fight off depression with a combination of supplementary vitamin B_6 and a lot of exercise. Physical exertion has been found to change brain chemistry and to promote a more optimistic attitude.

If this is not enough, you need someone to talk to. You should consult a clinical psychologist, a psychotherapist or a psychiatrist. Psychiatrists are medical doctors, who can prescribe drugs, whereas psychologists and psychotherapists may not have this right. To see a psychiatrist in private practice, you will need a referral from your regular health professional. The alternative is to use the Outpatient Psychiatric Services at your local hospital or speak to your nearest mental health association. Psychologists and many psychotherapists advertise; if you cannot or do not wish to get suggestions or referrals from friends or other health professionals, check with trained counselors at a nearby school or university. Counselors often know the best therapists in the community.

Whether you are dealing with a psychiatrist, psychologist, or psychotherapist, you should have some positive feelings about his or her competence and personality during the first visit. If not, try someone else.

You may also be offered medication either by your regular doctor, by a psychologist (working with a medical doctor), or by a psychiatrist. The first choice may be estrogen, although the *Physician's Desk Reference* tells us that "there is no adequate evidence that estrogens are effective for nervous symptoms or depression which might occur during menopause and they should not be used to treat these conditions."

It has been effectively demonstrated that menopause does not *cause* depression. What menopause may do is cause an intolerable amount of internal, physiological, and uncontrollable stress which, when added to the other stresses of midlife women, make it impossible to cope. The work of John and Sonja McKinlay, and of Susan Ballinger, clearly show that it is the *other* stresses that cause the problem. Estrogen therapy may be useful in a small minority of cases, perhaps because it relieves night sweats, allows a woman to sleep better, and thus enables her to cope with the other stresses. In the vast majority of cases, estrogen becomes a way to avoid dealing with problems aside from menopause.

The other "solution" available by prescription is tranquilizers, which will just make a woman more depressed. For authentic depression, antidepressants are preferable. They may stimulate the brain to produce its own "feel-good" chemicals to induce a more positive state of mind. The antidepressants may be bicyclic (Prozac), tricyclic or TCA (Elavil, Tofranil, etc.)—the drug of choice for many but causing major side effects (dry mouth, constipation, urinary retention) for some. If tricyclics cannot be tolerated, monoamine oxydase (MAO) inhibitors (Nardil or Parnate) may be substituted. MAO inhibitors cause severe headaches when taken with cheddar cheese, red wine, and a whole list of foods, beverages, and drugs. If you accept a prescription for an antidepressant, make sure you understand the anticipated effects of the medication, as well as the restrictions and possible side effects. If you can't get the information from anyone else, discuss it with your pharmacist.

Remember that depressions are self-limiting. Even if you choose *not* to accept medication, the counseling offered by a therapist may help you sort out how much of the current situation is due to menopause and how much may be due to other events going on in your life. Much of the horror of depression is self-induced, because many women feel that they don't *deserve* to be depressed. Rather than acknowledge the depression and deal with it, they stumble along—for six months or a year—hoping that it will just go away. It will, but it may be beneficial to help it along a little!

Sexual Functioning

Because sexual function is linked to both physical and psychological states, it deserves a place of its own. It is often said that the important question involving sex at menopause is not *how often?* but *with whom?* There are many women alone during menopause (divorced, widowed, or never married). For too many, sexual functioning becomes merely a decision about whether or not to masturbate.

For those women who *do* have partners, menopause may have a number of effects: intensity of both desire and response, increased desire but a slower response, infrequent or absence of desire with normal response when aroused, or decreased desire and response. From a psychological standpoint, such variation can be accounted for in a number of ways. A woman may experience the loss of reproductive ability as sexual freedom: desire and response may intensify. Another woman finds sexual activity enhanced by the risk of pregnancy: without the risk, desire wanes although she may still respond. Another woman has never enjoyed intercourse. Unless there is more time spent in undisturbed lovemaking or there are other positive changes (such as a new partner), both desire and response may disappear. It has been found that depressed women are more likely to dream about sex; like sex fantasies, sex dreams often translate into heightened desire. The possibilities are many.

I have been separated for over four years (with no intimacy for years before that) and, in the intervening time, have married off three of the four children who had remained at home, had a hysterectomy and a period of mild hot flashes. During a particularly stressful period, I had even developed what the doctor termed "senile vaginitis." What a dreadful term for a young lady of fifty-two! And then it happened—a "date" after thirty-five years. The friendship with this man, seven years my senior, turned into a full-blown romance and I couldn't believe my body's response! My hormones were dancing in double quick time and I don't remember anything as exciting as this even before age thirty-five. Here's to sex after fifty-three—it's wonderful!

Many women enter menopause with healthy levels of desire and response but, as they move into their fifties, they start to view *themselves* as less desirable. They find their bodies lacking—too fat, too flabby, too wrinkled; this may be a psychological concern but it may also take into account a real change in physical appearance. Some women find that any kind of romantic caressing triggers a hot flash, and this alone can diminish one's response to a sexual overture. Some find that they are suddenly extraordinarily sensitive to touch; rather than "turning them on," it causes them to flinch. This is very difficult to explain to a partner. Women who once anticipated many orgasms now find that they are satisfied with fewer, perhaps one or two, and that the orgasms are not so intense as they once were.

> I am fifty-one and ended my periods two years ago, have
> had hot sweats for five years but this is secondary
> to my real problem, which began two years ago. For
> some reason, it seems that this, the most devastating
> problem of my menopause—the abrupt end of any sexual
> pleasure—has received very little print. Although I
> had read several books, for some time I did not realize
> that my problem was midlife-related. My innermost feeling
> is one of rage. I feel cheated and at times find it very
> difficult to deal with. I can now realize why marriages
> end. My own mate is also my best friend so we are
> okay, but how I feel for women not so lucky!

Regular orgasm is known to be a precondition for a healthy vagina, and sexual activity (including masturbation) may help to prevent future problems which, as already mentioned, include vaginal changes. The vagina tends to shorten and the walls grow thinner as menopause proceeds. Lubrication takes longer, requiring more foreplay. One menopause study tells us that one-quarter of menopausal women will experience discomfort during intercourse about 50 percent of the time. Sexual activity is more likely to remain pleasurable when the woman has a measure of control over the depth of penetration (as, for instance, lying on or beside her partner) and the confidence to voice her needs.

Sex After Surgery

Women who have had surgery often have additional problems. Hysterectomized women may find that the quality of the orgasm changes, that the deep, inside-the-body feeling produced by a throbbing uterus is lamentably absent. Research suggests that orgasmic response may result from pressure-sensitive nerves in the cervix, which react to penile thrusting. In the absence of a cervix, the quality of the orgasm is bound to change. Many women who have lost a uterus and/or ovaries also report a complete absence of sexual arousal. Until recently, this was considered to be an individual and psychological response to surgery. Doctors assumed that women could only enjoy sex if they could make babies. It is now recognized that a fundamental physiological loss occurs in surgery, that the uterus itself may have important functions in *addition* to its acknowledged role as a "baby bag." It is important that women *know* that the amputation of sexual desire is neither intended nor foreseen. It is certainly not the woman's fault. This is just one more reason why hysterectomies and, above all, oophorectomies should be performed only after long and careful deliberation.

> I had a hysterectomy and partial oophorectomy at forty-three. The surgery left me a wreck. Although things were not great between my husband and me prior to the operation, the relationship took a nosedive largely because of my ensuing depression. I was teary and felt out of control. It took about a year for me to regain most of my former well-being. The biggest physical effect of the surgery has been the loss of desire for sex. Since my operation, my sex drive has lessened enormously. My husband and I are at a loss as to what to do.

If sexual function has been affected by surgery, there are avenues to be explored. If the problem is painful intercourse *(dyspareunia)*, most doctors are very willing to provide a prescription for estrogen cream. When hormones are not advisable, water-based lubricating jellies or products like Replens or Astroglide may make intercourse pleasurable once again. If the problem is absence of desire, your first step may be to establish credibility with your surgeon. For too many years, women have been told that absence of desire, or loss of libido, was an individual problem related to underlying feelings about sex *prior* to the operation. This is a no-win situation for a woman because it is impossible to prove what one's "underlying" feelings are about *anything*, and it is hard to make a convincing case about how one used to feel or act in bed. (This is compellingly described in the provocative book *The Castrated Woman* by Naomi Miller Stokes.)

Estrogen therapy rarely alleviates the loss of sexual desire, although it may make a woman feel better in other ways. ET tends to reduce the levels of circulating testosterone which, over time, may blunt the desire for sex. On the other hand, administration of male hormones may restore some or all of the missing sexual desire but, to be effective, this may have to be done within a short time of the surgery. The male hormone is variously described as an androgen or testosterone; testosterone is a form of androgen, a "male hormone" even though small amounts are produced in a normally functioning female—as is estrogen in a normally functioning male. Your gynecologist may be willing to read the relevant research and, if appropriate, prescribe for you. If the problem is the quality of the orgasm, or the need for extended foreplay (to aid lubrication), then a sex therapist might be a valuable ally.

Sex During Natural Menopause

If sexual function is problematic during a natural menopause, it is more likely to be a temporary situation. The traditional explanation is that women are mourning the loss of reproductive ability, and that this is unconsciously translated into a distaste for sex. Although this may be true for some women, it certainly is not true for the vast majority. More likely, the capacity for both desire and response will be affected by energy levels and feelings of self-esteem. Many women report an inability to experience intense feelings of sexual response. Those who are not fit may find that unusual exertion or orgasm may bring on a muscle spasm. Sexual difficulties arise in long-term relationships when we permit ourselves to draw invidious comparisons with "sex in the good old days," or when male partners—unwilling to admit that their own sex drive is not what it once was—blame lack of sexual activity on the women.

Women involved in *new* relationships report very few sexual problems during menopause; in fact, they often find that sex is better than ever. There are few studies of lesbian relationships during menopause, but those we have tell us that sexuality rarely deteriorates at this time of life, because nondemanding sex play is possible and mutually enjoyable. This suggests that strong bonds of affection and clear communication are crucial to mutually satisfactory sexual relationships during menopause. At one time, sexuality in the elderly was viewed as unnatural, even obscene. Today, sexuality in the middle-aged is seen as merely the continuation of sexuality in the thirties and forties. This may not be true, however. A fifty-year-old woman is not the same as a forty-year-old. There is very little research available on sex in the fifties. It's possible that it is different in both quality and quantity from sexual activity among younger adults.

REFERENCES AND RESOURCES

Ballinger, S. E. and W. L. Walker. *Not the Change of Life: Breaking the Menopause Taboo.* Ringwood, Australia: Penguin, 1987.

Ballinger, S. E. "A comparison of life stresses and symptomatology of menopause clinic patients and non-patients." Paper presented at the

4th International Congress on the Menopause, Buena Vista, Florida, 1984.

Barbach, L. and L. Levine. *Shared Intimacies: Women's Sexual Experiences.* NY: Bantam, 1980.

Bart, P. B. "Depression in middle-aged women," in *Woman in Sexist Society,* Gornick and Moran, eds., NY: Basic Books, 1971.

Belenky, M. F., B. M. Clinchy, N. R. Goldberger, and J. M. Tarule. *Women's Ways of Knowing: The Development of Self, Voice and Mind.* NY: Basic Books, 1986.

Channon, L. S. and S. E. Ballinger. "Some aspects of sexuality and vaginal symptoms during menopause and their relation to anxiety and depression," *British J. Med. Psychol., 59*:173–180, 1986.

Chesler, P. *Women and Madness.* NY: Doubleday, 1972.

Donovan, M. E. and L. T. Sanford. *Women & Self-Esteem.* NY: Doubleday, 1984.

Gillett, R. *Overcoming Depression: A Practical Self-Help Guide to Prevention and Treatment.* Toronto: Macmillan, 1988.

Johnson, K. "Women and depression," *Medical SelfCare,* 28:15, Spring 1985.

Kitzinger, S. *Woman's Experience of Sex.* NY: Putnam, 1983.

Lax, R. "The expectable depressive climacteric reaction," *Bulletin of the Menninger Clinic, 46*(2): 151–167, 1982.

Lerner, H. G. *The Dance of Anger.* NY: Harper & Row, 1985; and *The Dance of Intimacy.* NY: Harper & Row, 1989.

Lewisohn, P. M. et al. "Age at first onset for nonbipolar depression," *J. Abnormal Psychol., 95*(4):378–383, 1986.

Luria, Z. and R. G. Meade. "Sexuality and the Middle-aged Woman," *Women in Midlife,* Baruch and Brooks-Gunn, eds. NY: Plenum, 1984.

Mansfield, P. K., A. M. Voda, and P. B. Koch. "Midlife sexual response changes: Effects of menopausal transition & context." Unpublished.

Masters, W., V. Johnson, and R. Kolodny. *Human Sexuality* (2d ed.). Boston: Little, Brown, 1985.

Matthews, K. A., R. R. Wing, L. H. Kuller et al. "Influences of natural menopause on psychological characteristics and symptoms of middle-aged healthy women," *J. Consulting & Clin. Psychol., 58*(3):345–351, 1990.

McCann, L. and D. S. Holmes. "Influence of aerobic exercise on depression," *J. Pers. Soc. Psychol., 46*:1142–1147, 1984.

McCoy, N. L. and J. M. Davidson. "A longitudinal study of the effects of menopause on sexuality," *Maturitas, 17*:203–210, 1985.

McKinlay, J. B. and N. Bifano. "Does the menopause cause depression in normally aging women?" Paper presented to the Society for Epidemiological Research, Durham, NC, 1985.

Scarf, M. *Unfinished Business: Pressure Points in the Lives of Women.* NY: Doubleday, 1980.

Shainess, N. *Sweet Suffering.* NY: Wallaby Books, 1984.

Sherwin, B. B. "Changes in sexual behavior as a function of plasma sex steroid levels in postmenopausal women," *Maturitas,* 7:225, 1985.

Sherwin, B. B., M. M. Gelfand, and W. Brender. "Androgen enhances sexual motivation in females: A prospective, crossover study of sex steroid administration in the surgical menopause," *Psychosom. Med.,* 474:339–351, 1985.

Tannen, D. *You Just Don't Understand: Women and Men in Conversation.* NY: Morrow, 1990.

Tavris, C. *Anger: The Misunderstood Emotion.* NY: Simon & Schuster, 1982.

Women and Psychotherapy: A Consumer Handbook. Federation of Organizations for Professional Women (FOPW), 2000 P Street NW, Suite 403, Washington, DC 20036.

5

The Big Question: Hormones

As they approach menopause, many women worry about the hazards or benefits of estrogen therapy (ET) and combined hormone therapy (CHT), often without really understanding the issues. There is controversy about the reputed benefits of hormones before, during, and after menopause. Only a fraction of the controversy reaches the popular press. This is partially because of the complexity of the situation, and partially due to the enormous influence and power of the pharmaceutical companies and their views about what the public *needs* to know.

I was so appalled by the one-sided view of menopause (i.e., a deficiency syndrome requiring hormones for all or almost all women) presented at the 1991 meetings of the North American Menopause Society that I put together a presentation—slides and commentary—to guide women through the steps of making a decision about hormone therapy. There have been many inquiries about the availability of this presentation, some based on the hope that it's a slide/*tape* presentation that can easily be shipped off. But the intricacies and new developments make such a decision-making process too complex to be permanently recorded on tape. The situation is in flux and last-minute information must be accommodated. Therefore it remains a presentation to be made in person. It is with some trepidation that I attempt to summarize that presentation in this chapter. Who knows what tomorrow may bring?

We are in a unique situation in this country. It is the only country in the world (with the exception perhaps of Canada) where gynecologists are so frequently primary physicians. In the countries of Western Europe, most women see a family physician (in some cases, *must* see a family physician) before they see a gynecologist. Gynecologists specialize in reproductive organs and are trained surgeons whereas family physicians are more interested in other aspects of the patient's life and are more likely to consider other events or situations that might have an impact on her experience of menopause.

Here in America, the pharmaceutical companies concentrate their sales efforts on gynecologists because these doctors write twice as many prescriptions for hormone therapy than family physicians. (For instance, hysterectomies are almost always performed by gynecologists, and women who've had hysterectomies use five times more hormone prescriptions than do naturally menopausal women.) Most doctors are too busy to research the claims and counterclaims of different drug manufacturers. They are influenced by the avalanche of publicity about hormones—advertisements in medical journals, reprints of research studies brought to their offices by pharmaceutical representatives—in addition to the luncheons, dinners, conferences, and meetings sponsored, funded, or supported by drug companies.

To balance this one-sided view, many women and women's groups continue to publish articles, newsletters, and books stressing the other side of the story—potential side effects, the possibility of long-term adverse effects and, most of all, the absence of properly designed studies of menopausal hormones.

The issues are complex but, even so, these are important concerns for women at midlife and it is essential that they keep themselves informed.

What Hormones Are

Although a great deal is known about hormones in the body, there still remains much that is not known. Hormones are produced primarily by endocrine (ductless) glands, which means that the hormones produced are pumped directly into the bloodstream. Doctors who specialize in the study of hormones are called endocrinologists. They are the first to acknowledge that the glands of the female reproductive system operate in an intricate manner still only partially understood.

When we talk about estrogen produced inside the body (endogenous estrogen), we usually mean a particular kind of estrogen from the ovaries called estradiol (estra-DY-ol). This is not the only form of estrogen in the body. Both the ovaries and the adrenal glands (perched on the kidneys) produce substances that are converted to another form of estrogen, estrone. Estrone, which is instrumental in producing strong bone, is produced in very small amounts during the reproductive years, but assumes more importance during menopause and postmenopause. A third kind of estrogen is also present—estriol, formed by the interaction of estradiol and estrone.

The process of estradiol production is initiated by the hypothalamus, a small gland in the brain. This gland, in turn, stimulates the nearby pituitary gland to produce FSH (follicle-stimulating hormone) and LH (luteinizing hormone), together known as gonadotropins. A follicle is the small vessel inside the ovary that contains an ovum, or egg. Stimulated by the FSH, the follicle begins to produce estradiol, the major estrogen of the menstruating years. This hormone ensures a buildup of cells within the uterus (or womb) to provide a safe environment for a fertilized egg. A high level of estradiol in the blood signals the pituitary to decrease FSH production and to send out LH instead.

MAJOR GLANDS AND REPRODUCTIVE ORGANS

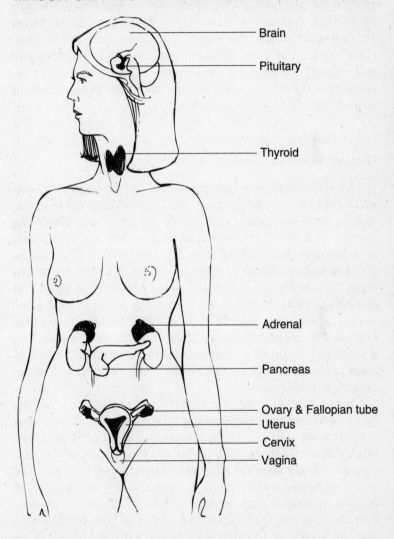

Brain

Pituitary

Thyroid

Adrenal

Pancreas

Ovary & Fallopian tube
Uterus
Cervix
Vagina

LH causes the follicle to burst producing an egg; this process is called *ovulation.* The egg travels into the fallopian tube while the spent follicle transforms itself into a *corpus luteum* (yellow body), which produces progesterone, the hormone that opposes or counteracts the effects of estrogen. Progesterone takes over during the latter part of the menstrual cycle (the days between ovulation and menstruation) and, should the egg *not* be fertilized, the progesterone ensures that the lining of the uterus (the endometrial tissue) is flushed out during menstruation.

Natural Hormone Changes at Menopause

As one approaches menopause, the follicle may take longer to rupture, requiring more FSH, a higher level of estradiol in the bloodstream, and a thicker layer of cells inside the uterus. As a result, menstruation may be late and may result in a heavier than normal flow. A high level of FSH in the blood is one indication of menopausal onset and is one of the signs that doctors look for when doing hormonal assays to establish menopausal status. (Although the assay is most often part of a standard "one-shot" blood test, reliable results require a series of tests through one day and over a period of a month.) By the time a hormonal assay confirms imminent menopause, most women are already well aware that a major change is underway.

Many women react to high levels of FSH by feeling "blue" and by temporarily losing interest in sex. This is characteristic not only of premenopause but also of the time just after childbirth, when high levels of FSH stimulate the first regular menstrual cycle after many months without periods.

It may take weeks, months, or years, but eventually the ovaries no longer produce eggs or follicles. Estradiol production declines, but the ovaries' production of both testosterone and the precursor to estrone increases with age. Because estrone is formed from substances produced by both ovaries

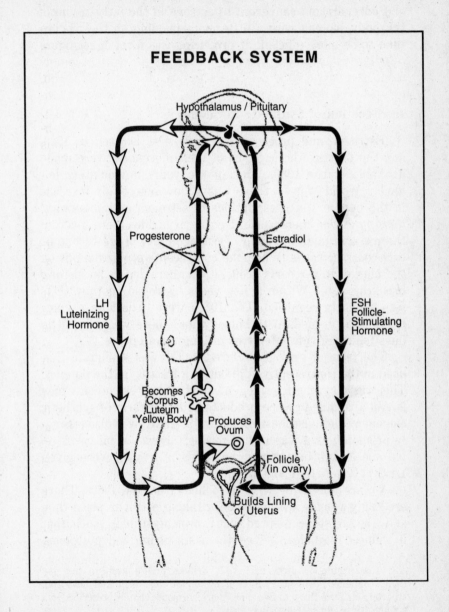

FEEDBACK SYSTEM

Hypothalamus / Pituitary

Progesterone

Estradiol

LH
Luteinizing
Hormone

FSH
Follicle-
Stimulating
Hormone

Becomes
Corpus
Luteum
"Yellow Body"

Produces
Ovum

Follicle
(in ovary)

Builds Lining
of Uterus

and adrenals and converted to estrone in the fatty tissue of the body, women with a little more padding on their bones tend to be more efficient at producing this form of estrogen.

Introduction of Synthetic Hormones

Estrogen and progesterone were first isolated in 1923, and the first synthetic forms of these hormones were made available in the 1930s. During the years immediately following World War II, there was a slow but steady increase in the numbers of prescriptions of estrogen as *replacement therapy* during menopause. Enormous strides were made in the use and understanding of estrogen and progesterone as oral contraceptives. When the contraceptive pill was put on the market in the early 1960s, it was heralded as an historic breakthrough.* Within a few years, estrogen therapy (ET) was similarly regarded. The 1960s were a decade of enormous faith in medical technology, and there was very little questioning of side effects or of long-term effects.

The form of estrogen offered in ET was similar to that used in the contraceptive pill but at a fraction of the potency. This was a synthetic estrogen called ethinyl estradiol, which is still available in some products. Another form of synthetic estrogen (diethylstilbestrol, known as DES) was also strongly promoted as a way of minimizing the risk of miscarriage. No one knows how many thousands of women were given DES between 1941 and 1971.

We are still living with the fallout from the 1960s. There are many women who have been taking estrogen since then and who are still convinced that it prolonged their youth, that it reduced wrinkles, helped them stay slim, and postponed

*The formulation of this early "pill" delivered more hormones in a day than is contained in a month's supply of the new low-dose form. And today's pill still contains from three to five times more hormones than is prescribed in a standard dose of menopausal hormones.

graying of the hair. In fact, all these claims for estrogen—
once widely believed—have been found to be false.

After the initial infatuation with the pill, drawbacks began
to be noticed—including an enormously increased risk of heart
attack for women in their forties (most of them smokers). In
response to concerns about these synthetic hormones, a new
form of conjugated estrogen was developed, more nearly re-
sembling human estrogen. This conjugated estrogen is estrone,
rather than estradiol. Because it is collected from animals (Premarin, a trademark of Wyeth-Ayerst, is derived from *pregnant
mares' urine*), it is often referred to as "natural" rather than
"synthetic." This really means that the chemical composition of
the estrogen more nearly corresponds to human estrogen.

Recent History of Hormone Use

From 1965 to 1975, menopausal estrogen was one of the
four most commonly prescribed drugs in North America. It
was believed that estrogen was a "youth" drug, that it kept
women slim, unlined, and youthful. Then, in 1971, it was discovered that DES caused malformations and sometimes disease in the reproductive organs of babies born to mothers
who took DES. (It is now known that these children are six
times more likely to be infertile and that the mothers themselves are also at significantly increased risk of breast cancer.)
Following this tragic discovery, it was found that the rates of
endometrial cancer for women taking *menopausal* estrogens
was somewhere between six and fourteen times the norm,
with the increase in risk dependent on duration and strength
of the daily dose. Moreover, the increased risk remained for
at least ten years after estrogen was discontinued.

The sales of estrogens plummeted after this revelation.
At the same time, research projects multiplied in a frantic
attempt to find ways to make estrogen more safe.

Estrogen, when not "opposed" by progesterone as in the
normal cycle (see page 88) stimulates the growth of cells in the
uterus. When these cells are not washed away in a monthly

menstrual period, the thickness and depth of the endometrium (lining of the uterus) can set the stage for a slow-growing cancer. Fortunately, it is a type of cancer that, if caught in time, is 97 percent curable—but at the price of a hysterectomy. (Choosing to take estrogen without progesterone, and to incur the risk of a hysterectomy, is not recommended. See chapter 7.)

A standard Pap test cannot detect endometrial cancer, so a woman who is on estrogen therapy, and who has a uterus should have an endometrial biopsy every six months. This procedure is somewhat like a D&C, using a cell sampler or a more recent innovation that uses a small-caliber, flexible plastic system that can be inserted through the cervix and into the uterus. A sample of cells is then suctioned out for analysis. If the physician is experienced with this procedure, false negatives (mistaken judgments that nothing is amiss) are substantially reduced. The newer suction curettes are more comfortable and avoid some of the pain during, and severe cramping following, the use of standard cell samplers. Women are told that the procedure is momentarily uncomfortable, but many women find the experience too painful to accept as a semi-annual necessity.

The alternative to routine endometrial biopsy is to add progesterone to the estrogen therapy (making combined hormone therapy, or CHT) to mimic the natural cycle of hormones. This practice has become so widespread that estrogens have more than made up for the dip in sales between 1975 and 1985. In 1990, estrogen enjoyed unparalleled popularity and was outsold only by one prescription medication appropriate for *both* men and women.

How Estrogen is Prescribed

Premarin tablets and the Estraderm patch are the most commonly prescribed forms of menopausal estrogen in North America. The Premarin tablet is available in five strengths— .3 mg, .625 mg, .9 mg, 1.25 mg, and 2.5 mg. The Estraderm patch (manufactured by Ciba-Geigy) is sold in two sizes and strengths—50 mcg and 100 mcg—and is applied twice a week on the thigh, buttock, or abdomen. The tablet is less expensive than the patch, but the estrogen in the tablet must be metabolized by the liver, which makes the patch more appropriate for women with a tendency to liver disease or to high blood pressure. About 30 percent of women who try the patch react badly to the adhesive and must discontinue it.

Other forms of estrogen are available in pill form to be taken orally (Ogen, Estrace, TACE) or placed under the tongue to dissolve, in vaginal creams, in injections, in pellets (surgically implanted under the top layer of skin on the abdomen or inner thigh), in a vaginal ring (inserted and left in place to slowly deliver estrogen into the system), in a gel (rubbed into the skin of the abdomen), and in combination pills similar to oral contraceptive pills. A patch that combines estrogen and progestins may also be available soon, but this patch, as well as the pellets, vaginal ring, gel, and combination pills are not yet approved for use in this country. Some are synthetic forms of estrogen, similar to that used in the oral contraceptive (e.g., Estinyl, Estrovis), whereas others are the more "natural" form (i.e., Premarin, Estrace, Estratab, Ogen).

Synthetic progesterones (progestins or progestogens) are available in two basic types: one, medroxyprogesterone, is progesterone-based; the other, the norethindrone type, is more androgenic, which means it affects the body as male hormones do. Progestins often provoke side effects, but medroxyprogesterone (used in Provera) is more easily tolerated. Commonly prescribed are Provera tablets (from Upjohn), available in 2.5 mg, 5 mg, and 10 mg. Norlutate is an example of an androgenic progestin. (Although it is widely prescribed, no progestin has ever been approved by the FDA for the treatment of menopause.)

Natural progesterone is used by some physicians (who have it made up by a pharmacist), which is a welcome trend because of the reduced side effects as compared to synthetic progestins. Some women are also using a progesterone-based moisturizing cream derived from discorea (wild yam); prelim-

SOME COMMON

Drug Name	Active Ingredients	Size
ESTINYL Oral Tablet	*Ethinyl estradiol*	0.02 mg
		0.05 mg
ESTRACE Oral Tablet	*Estradiol*	1 mg
		2 mg
ESTRACE Vaginal Cream	*Estradiol*	0.1 mg in 1 g of cream
ESTRADERM Transdermal Patch (box of 8)	*Estradiol*	4 mg = 0.05 mg/day 8 mg = 0.1 mg/day
ESTRATEST H.S. Oral Tablet	*Esterified estrogens Methyltestosterone*	.625 mg 1.25 mg
ESTRATEST Oral Tablet	*Esterified estrogens Methyltestosterone*	1.25 mg 2.5 mg
MENRIUM Oral Tablet	*Esterified estrogens Chlordiazepoxide (tranquilizer)*	0.4 mg 10 mg
OGEN Oral Tablet	*Estropipate*	.625 mg
		1.5 mg
		3 mg
		6 mg
OGEN Vaginal Cream	*Estropipate*	1.5 mg in 1 g of cream
PREMARIN Oral Tablet (package of 25)	*Conjugated equine estrogens*	0.3 mg
		.625 mg
		0.9 mg
		1.25 mg
		2.5 mg
PREMARIN Vaginal Cream	*Conjugated estrogen*	.625 mg in 1 g of cream
PREMARIN + Methyltestosterone Oral Tablet	*Conjugated estrogens Methyltestosterone*	.625 mg 5 mg
	Conjugated estrogens Methyltestosterone	1.25 mg 10 mg
PMB 200 Oral Tablet	*Conjugated estrogens Meprobamate (tranquilizer)*	.45 mg 200 mg
PMB 400 Oral Tablet	*Conjugated estrogens Meprobamate (tranquilizer)*	.45 mg 400 mg

MENOPAUSAL ESTROGENS

Color	Dosage	Contains	
		lactose	tartrazine
buff	0.02 to 0.05 mg daily	X	X
pink		X	
lavender	Initial 1 or 2 mg daily.	X	
turquoise	Maintenance at 0.5 mg to 20 mg	X	X
	2 to 4 g daily for 1 or 2 weeks, then reduce to ½ dosage for similar period. Maintenance at 1 to 3 g weekly		
10 cm² round 20 cm² oblong	Affix to abdomen. Change twice weekly on same days every week. Take with a minimum of 10 days progestins, every month or 3 months, to protect uterus.		
dark green	One or two daily cyclically	X	
light green	One or two daily cyclically	X	
purple	Three times daily cyclically Addictive		
yellow		X	X
peach	Twice daily	X	
blue		X	
lime		X	
	2 to 4 g daily		
green	One daily for 25 days (cyclic)	X	
maroon		X	
pink	or	X	
yellow	One daily (continuous) with progestins	X	
purple		X	
	2 to 4 g daily cyclically to start		
white	One or two daily for 25 days		
yellow	One or two daily for 25 days		
green	Three times daily cyclically Addictive	X	
pink	Three times daily cyclically Addictive	X	

MENOPAUSAL PROGESTINS

DRUG	ACTIVE INGREDIENTS	SIZE
AMEN Oral Tablet	*Medroxyprogesterone acetate*	10 mg
AYGESTIN Oral Tablet	*Norethindrone acetate*	5 mg
CYCRIN Oral Tablet	*Medroxyprogesterone acetate*	10 mg
NATURAL PROGESTERONE Capsules or Vaginal Suppository		25 mg
		50 mg
		100 mg
		200 mg
NORLUTATE Oral Tablet	*Norethindrone acetate*	5 mg
NORLUTIN Oral Tablet	*Norethindrone*	5 mg
PROVERA Oral Tablet	*Medroxyprogesterone acetate*	2.5 mg
		5 mg
		10 mg

Interesting points:
- Many pills contain **lactose,** which may be difficult to digest.
- Many pills contain **tartrazine** (Yellow No. 5 dye) to which many aspirin-sensitive people are allergic.
- Degree of atrophy affects level of estrogen cream absorption.
- Severe cases of atrophy should start with 10 days/1.25 mg oral therapy for conditioning.
- Oral prescription should be adjusted according to estrogen cream absorption levels.

AND PROGESTERONE

COLOR	DOSAGE	CONTAINS	
		lactose	tartrazine
layered peach & white	5 to 10 mg day for 5–10 days, beginning on 16th day of cycle. Bleeding starts 3rd to 7th day after stopping	?	?
oblong white	2.5 mg to 10 mg for 5–10 days	X	
oval peach	5 to 10 mg day for 5–10 days, beginning on 16th day of cycle. Bleeding starts 3rd to 7th day after stopping	X	
	Made up by pharmacist following physician's directions. 100 mg twice daily		
pink, cup-shaped	2.5 to 10 mg from 5th to 25th day of cycle	X	X
white, cup-shaped	5 to 20 mg from 5th to 25th day of cycle		
orange	daily continuously or twice daily cyclically	X	X
hexagonal white	5 to 10 mg daily for 10–12 days, beginning	X	
round white	Day 13 or 15 of cycle	X	

- **Possible side effects of estrogen include:**
  cystitis-like syndrome, premenstrual-like syndrome, skin rashes, spots, pimples, or blisters, hirsutism (body hair), intolerance to contact lenses, migraine, dizziness, headache, depression, reduced carbohydrate tolerance, changes in libido, thinning hair.
- **Possible side effects of progestins include:**
  backache, insomnia, dizziness, nervousness, somnolence.
- **Possible side effects of methyltestosterone include:** reduced carbohydrate tolerance, clitoral enlargement (which is usually not reversible when drug is discontinued), lower voice, hirsutism, frontal hair loss, anxiety, depression, burning, prickling, formication.

inary studies claim that it will protect against both bone loss
and menopausal symptoms. If proven effective, this could be
a very comfortable way to absorb progesterone.

The most common regimen (method of administration)
prescribed in this country specifies Premarin (commonly .625
mg) daily for days 1 through 25 of the month* *or* an
Estraderm patch for 3½ weeks (7 patches). Progestins (usually Provera at 5 mg) are added between days 14 through 25.
Then both the estrogen and progestin are withdrawn and a
bleed takes place. In postmenopause, this monthly bleed may
diminish and eventually disappear. (If another form of estrogen is used, the cyclic regimen may specify 21 days of medication and 7 days of no medication.)

In response to many complaints about the prolongation of
monthly periods when using this regimen (coupled with some
annoying side effects of Provera—headaches, sore breasts,
etc.), some physicians are permitting their patients to use
the progestins only every third, or even every sixth month.
The point is to have a regular withdrawal bleed to shed the
excess cells stimulated by estrogen in the endometrium.
(This is obviously unnecessary for a woman who has had a
hysterectomy.)

Another way of avoiding the monthly bleed is to use both
hormones on a continuous basis. This continuous combined
therapy usually involves taking Premarin daily, accompanied
by the lowest possible dose (2.5 mg) of Provera. Ideally, this
should eliminate bleeding entirely, although it will not confer
the benefits to blood fats of the cyclical regimen (see page
143). Moreover, many women experience episodes of breakthrough bleeding on this regimen. This may resolve over
time—after approximately six months. However, many wom-

*Day 1 of a menstrual cycle is counted from the day of the appearance
of menstruation. In the absence of a menstrual cycle, Day 1 is usually the
first day of the calendar month. This is to make it easier for the woman and
her doctor to remember. However, if the withdrawal bleed is inconvenient
at the end of the month, Day 1 can be arbitrarily fixed at any day of the
month, provided this is consistent.

en find it easier to tolerate the predictable bleeds of the older, cyclic regimen.

Who Can or Can't Take Hormones?

Estrogen and progestins, alone or separately, have profound effects on the body, and it is not clear exactly how progestins modify the effects of estrogen. High estrogen levels in the bloodstream have been associated with elevated blood pressure (hypertension) and blood clots (thromboembolisms or phlebitis), although the precise relationship is not clearly understood. Women who take oral estrogen are more than twice as likely to require gallstone surgery; creams and patches don't carry this risk. Some of these negative effects have been traced to oral contraceptives that contain synthetic estrogens and, as mentioned earlier, at much higher doses than is normal for menopausal ET. But because it was not known whether it was the form of estrogen, or the amount, menopausal ET was, until recently, either not prescribed at all or prescribed reluctantly to menopausal women with a tendency to blood clots, gallbladder disease, or high blood pressure, *or* to women with a family or personal history of cancer. (Estrogen is known to stimulate certain types of breast tumors, primarily the estrogen-dependent type characteristic of younger, premenopausal women.)

Uterine fibroids thrive in the presence of estrogen, and women with fibroids who experience pressure, pain, or heavy bleeding often notice welcome relief of symptoms with the naturally occurring reduction of estrogen at menopause. Therefore, women with fibroids should avoid ET if at all possible.

Much to my surprise my doctor prescribed estrogen for depression. At the same time, he asked me if I knew that I had many large fibroids. I told him I *did* know and asked what their effect would be. He told me that

they would cause erratic periods but made absolutely
no mention of any other possible problems. Luckily,
I had been on the ET for only six weeks before I read
that estrogen would enlarge fibroids. I haven't taken
estrogen since and find that exercise and vitamins keep
the depression at bay as well as ET ever did.

Because obese women (i.e., women who are more than 20
percent over ideal weight) tend to produce a lot of estrone as
a result of their large numbers of fat cells, those who are put
on ET should be closely monitored.

Reasons for Prescribing Hormone Therapy

Most women complain of some kinds of menopausal effects during the period of time when estradiol levels decline
and estrone production increases (see page 88). Hot flashes
are the most common complaint, and estrogen alleviates hot
flashes for most women.

We still don't know exactly what causes a flash. A surge
of LH has been noted to occur at the same time as a hot
flash, but there is some other mechanism at work that hasn't
yet been established. The flash may be caused by a *fall* in estrogen, suggesting that hot flashes may be due more to sudden changes in estrogen levels rather than, as commonly
believed, the lack of estrogen. Adding estrogen from outside
the body may alleviate hot flashes, but may also postpone adjustment to new levels and new kinds of estrogen from inside
the body.

When ET or CHT is prescribed to alleviate hot flashes,
the usual recommendation is to take the lowest possible dose
for the shortest possible time.

Estrogen is often prescribed to relieve depression even
though this is effective for only a small minority of women
(see chapter 4). An interesting report from Britain notes that
women on estrogen are more than twice as likely to commit

suicide as those who don't use estrogen. This reflects the problem of inappropriate use of estrogen for women who are deeply depressed; hormone use does not solve the underlying problem. The stresses that contribute to depression are too often ignored.

> I am fifty years old and had a total hysterectomy at the
> age of thirty-three. Since then I've been taking ET
> and have now discovered that, although the side
> effects are worsening, I am unable to get along without
> it. The most unusual of these side effects is a great sensation
> of heat on my left side. Besides this, my face and
> breasts swell, I'm continuously short of breath, and
> my legs ache. I attempted to go off estrogen for a month
> and, although the side effects disappeared, I found myself
> getting terrible hot flashes and sinking into a terrible
> depression. I am now taking "nerve pills" prescribed
> by the doctor. Unfortunately, he has not been helpful
> in explaining how I could wean myself off the estrogen.

There is a very real concern that estrogen produces a psychological and physical dependence that some women find difficult to break. We hear from many women who are discontinuing use of hormones for a variety of reasons. Usually, the doctor has recommended it but has not been very helpful about how to do so. We counsel women to reduce the estrogen very slowly, either by obtaining a prescription for a lower dose or by cutting tablets in half or in quarters, or by taking it every second or third day so that the body can gradually adjust to lower levels. When using the patch, she can cut it in half or thirds, tape the open edges closed, and apply as usual. Hot flashes may return for some time and may be very uncomfortable, but this is usually a temporary rebound effect. Eventually the body adjusts to the lower level of estrogen characteristic of postmenopause.

Although estrogen causes the skin to retain more moisture, and the slight swelling sometimes makes fine wrinkles less visible, estrogen does not prevent wrinkles. For women with very fine, transparent skin, estrogen helps maintain a cushion of collagen under the outer layer of skin, adding a degree of firmness.

Estrogen may also relieve cystitis (the sensation of burning during urination) and other complaints of the vaginal/urinary system, including dry vagina. (See chapter 2 for more about estrogen cream.)

Estrogen is often prescribed for women who experience a loss of sex drive after reproductive surgery. Sometimes this is helpful because it compensates for the sudden loss of vaginal lubrication during sexual arousal, and it may also help restore sensitivity to the nipples. But women who have experienced oophorectomy lose the minute amounts of testosterone that contribute not only to libido (the desire for sex), but which appear also to influence a global sense of well-being. For these women, the addition of testosterone may make a big difference. The problem is that testosterone is difficult to control: even in slight overdoses, it can cause acne, enlarged clitoris, a more masculine (lower) voice, unwanted body hair—and it may very well contribute to an increased risk of heart disease.

Since 1985, both ET and CHT have been widely promoted as a way to prevent both osteoporosis and cardiovascular disease. In both cases, the hormone therapy is prolonged and serious questions arise about the advisability of putting *most* women on hormone therapy in order to protect only those at risk. More information about osteoporosis and cardiovascular disease is available in chapter 6. Here, we will examine the benefits and drawbacks of using hormones.

Exactly how estrogen functions to halt the loss of bone that culminates in osteoporosis is not completely understood, although it is known that estrogen stimulates the release of calcitonin, a hormone from the thyroid gland. Calcitonin, in turn, stops the release of bone tissue into the bloodstream. We know that women who have had a number of pregnancies (during which estrogen levels soar) are less vulnerable to osteoporosis, as are women who are overweight. (Some of this may be due to the benefits of the extra weight putting stress on bone; some may result from the higher production of estrone.) On the other hand, women who have their ovaries removed begin to experience bone loss immediately after surgery, and this bone loss proceeds more swiftly than in normally menopausal women (see chapter 6).

There is no doubt that estrogen is a valuable medication for women at risk. There is also no doubt that the numbers of women at risk are enormously inflated as a result of the vast number of hysterectomies, and particularly oophorectomies, which are performed in this country. Healthy ovaries are routinely and unnecessarily removed from women over forty—putting them at enormously increased risk of osteoporosis *and* cardiovascular disease.

A year and a half ago, I had a hysterectomy and oophorectomy. I was started on estrogen and progesterone and had bowel failure. The estrogen was taken away and my bowels started to function. The gynecologist I was seeing gave me hormone injections (estrogen plus testosterone) and another kind of synthetic estrogen over the course of about five months. I was then sent to an endocrinologist about the thirty-five pounds I had gained. His advice was to take a tranquilizer and stop worrying.

I went back to my family doctor really upset. I thought I was going off the deep end. I was having severe hot flashes, feeling depressed, suffering from severe anxiety, and had lost almost all interest in sex. He sent me to another endocrinologist who did a complete workup and found elevated levels of testosterone. He put me back on estrogen tablets, which did not help.

Lately, I've stopped taking the estrogen and progesterone. My body is now readjusting and finally I feel in control of myself and of my body.

Estrogen supplementation is currently being strongly promoted as a form of protection against cardiovascular disease, largely based on the results of a massive study of nurses, initially involving 122,000 married female registered nurses who were between thirty and fifty-five when the study began in 1976. These nurses have been followed at two-year intervals since and, in 1991, it was found that, based on ten years of data on 48,470 postmenopausal women, those taking estrogen were found to be at significantly decreased risk for major coronary disease.

Prior to this study, it was thought that women taking estrogen were probably healthier than women not taking estrogen, for a number of reasons. First, women taking estrogen are under the continuing care of a physician and must be willing to pay for monthly medication. Such women are likely to be in a higher-income bracket than women not on estrogen. We know that they are much more likely to be getting regular cholesterol checks, Pap smears, rectal exams, and mammograms. In addition, women with particular health problems—such as high blood pressure, diabetes, phlebitis, gallstones, history of cancer—were less likely to be prescribed estrogen.

Therefore, many of the claims that women on estrogen looked and felt better could be countered by the observation that women on estrogen had *always* looked and felt better, because only healthy women were taking estrogen. It was just not a valid comparison.

What the Nurses' Health Study has done is to supply enough information to offset this bias; in other words, to make valid comparisons between well-matched groups of women who do or don't take estrogens.

Estrogen, more specifically "natural" estrogen in tablet form, has the ability to increase blood levels of high density lipoproteins (HDL) by 10 to 15 percent, the importance of which is explained in the next chapter. It is clear that certain women *will* benefit and benefit markedly from this added protection against cardiovascular disease (CVD). But it is still not known just which women will benefit. There are lingering concerns about the tendency of some forms of estrogen to substantially increase the level of triglycerides (a kind of fat) in the blood. High levels of triglycerides seem to increase the risk of heart disease, particularly for women over fifty. This aspect of estrogen's effects needs more study. Moreover, estrogen provokes a sudden increase in blood pressure in some hypertensive women. Blood pressure soars, incurring threat of a stroke. (One woman in twenty with high blood pressure reacts in this way.) If estrogen is now seen to be protective against heart disease, how will these women fare?

The results of the Nurses' Health Study are based on women who were prescribed ET alone. The benefits of protection against cardiovascular disease are predicated on the basis of oral "natural" tablets only. For women who have a uterus and who want the additional protection of progestins against endometrial cancer, this is a real dilemma. Preliminary reports suggest that the addition of some progestins dilutes the positive effects of estrogen on HDLs in the blood. The good news is that, with natural micronized progesterone (which can be made up by a pharmacist under instructions from the prescribing physician), the increase in HDLs is virtually unchanged. Unfortunately, natural micronized progesterone is not widely known and thus is not yet easily available.

Medroxyprogesterone (Provera), which is both widely known and widely available, modifies somewhat the positive effects of estrogen on HDLs; to compensate, some physicians are ordering reduced doses of progestins and/or increased doses of estrogen. When a nortestosterone progestin (e.g., Norlutate) is prescribed, it may cancel out the benefits of ET on blood fats. There is a pronounced trend to lower doses of progestins to offset these effects, and the consensus is that low-dose progestin should be given for longer periods— twelve to fourteen days each month—to allow estrogen to work properly. It also means that the continuous combined regimen (outlined on page 98) is not considered protective against cardiovascular disease and that forms of estrogen other than natural oral tablets will need reevaluation.

Potential Side Effects of ET and CHT

One of the major concerns with both ET and CHT is noncompliance—that is, women who receive a prescription and never have it filled, or who have it filled but who start then stop taking the pills (or using the patch) as they wish. One study of 301 women who had been prescribed hormones noted that only 30 percent ever took the medication. Noncompliance is a major problem in evaluating the effectiveness of ET and/or CHT, but it is an aspect of hormone use that is consistently ignored.

Linked to this problem of noncompliance is the issue of side effects. Hormones are powerful medications and, in the effort to produce standardized dosages, the very individual reactions of many women are ignored or discounted. Estrogen therapy alone has been known to cause increased appetite; bloat; headaches; swollen, tender breasts; nausea; vomiting; cramps; dizziness; fluid retention; rashes; visual disturbances; depression; or changes in levels of sexual desire (libido). Some of these side effects may be eliminated by adjusting (usually reducing) the dose; but some may not. Estrogen may also cause breakthrough bleeding, which means bleeding between the expected times of menstrual bleeds.

Progestins (alone or in CHT) often cause swollen breasts, water retention, headaches, decreased sex drive, fatigue, and increased appetite.

Moreover, there is considerable evidence that ET may contribute to an increased risk of breast cancer. Preliminary data from Sweden suggest that this risk is increased with the addition of progestins in CHT, but we are awaiting confirmation.

The association of estrogen use and breast cancer remains speculative but there is evidence that long-term use (for ten years or more) can increase risk. Of more than forty-four studies on ET and breast cancer, some found significant increases in some subgroups of women while others found significant decreases in other subgroups. The cancer risks posed by progestins (CHT) remain speculative as well; their effect on the breast in particular is a matter of controversy and has not been the subject of adequate investigation.

—Office of Technology Assessment, *The Menopause, Hormone Therapy and Women's Health,* 40:1992

How to Make a Decision

The continuing controversy over risks and benefits of estrogen (ET) and estrogen-plus-progesterone (CHT) makes it difficult (but not impossible) for the individual woman to make an informed choice.

If menopause is viewed as a deficiency disease, or condition, as it is by some medical practitioners, then it follows that some kind of treatment will be viewed as beneficial to *all* women approaching menopause. If menopause is seen as a natural stage of biological development, however, estrogen will be seen as medication useful for those most seriously affected (i.e., those who have had an artificial menopause, those at serious risk of cardiovascular disease or osteoporosis, and those few women who suffer an intolerable menopause).

Some people feel that drugs were invented to cushion us from discomfort and stress, and that to spurn such relief is silly. Others believe that we swallow too many drugs without thinking of the consequences, and that sound nutrition and other changes in daily routine should be adopted before resorting to drugs. These differing attitudes influence many decisions about ET.

When a woman is prescribed ET (or CHT), it should follow a thorough medical examination, including not only blood pressure, pelvic exam, and a Pap smear, but also a measurement of blood lipids, a breast examination and mammogram and, ideally, a bone density scan. Her doctor will usually insist on a checkup in three months, and then every six months thereafter. This means that women on ET or CHT are *more* likely to have regular medical checkups than women not receiving estrogen. Because of this consistent surveillance, including endometrial biopsies, Pap tests, and breast exams, if they *do* develop signs of disease, it is more likely to be caught early.

Thus if a woman no longer has functioning ovaries, and particularly if the loss of ovaries occurs before the normal age of menopause, ET is probably a wise decision. If loss of sex drive results from oophorectomy, ET with added testosterone may be the only effective therapy. When the ovaries are removed, the uterus is usually removed as well: where there is no uterus, there is no worry about endometrial cancer. Given the enormously increased risks of osteoporosis and cardiovascular disease to women who go through early menopause as a result of surgery, ET is probably a wise move. (It is also worth noting that oophorectomy significantly reduces the risk of breast cancer.)

Similarly, because any form of premature menopause increases the risk of osteoporosis and perhaps of cardiovascular disease as well, women who go through an early menopause for any reason should seriously consider ET or CHT.

On the other hand, we have little to no information about the protective effects of a healthy lifestyle—regular vigorous exercise, no smoking, no or little alcohol, a low-fat, high-fiber diet. It's quite possible that these plusses would more than make up for the loss of ovaries. We just don't know.

Women who go through natural menopause but who find hot flashes, night sweats, or associated discomforts absolutely intolerable may choose to take CHT. This is a quality-of-life choice and should be respected. There is no evidence that CHT for a period of less than ten years increases the risk of breast cancer. Some women find that a short course of ET, or CHT, allows them to overcome the fatigue and emotional stress that makes decision making impossible. Once they are back on their feet, they can decide whether to continue with hormone therapy or to make other changes in their lives that may help them withstand the stresses of menopause. I've heard from women in high-powered jobs, or in the public eye, who have chosen to take hormones in their fifties in order to minimize the discomforts of menopause but who intend to wean themselves off the medication very slowly in the privacy of their well-deserved retirement years.

> There is no official standard or protocol for administering or prescribing CHT. Furthermore, no conclusive studies have been performed that indicate which regimen is most beneficial, and there have been no studies that meet design, duration, and sample size requirements for determining conclusively the risks and benefits of long-term use of CHT.
> —OTA, *The Menopause, Hormone*
> *Therapy and Women's Health,* 69:1992

Women who are at particular risk for osteoporosis have a more difficult choice to make, because they must embark on long-term ET or CHT to preserve their bones. They can roughly assess the situation for themselves (using the Osteoporosis Risk Profile in the next chapter) and verify this with results from a bone scan. They may decide to try vigorous exercise and be tested again. If estrogen is contraindicated for some reason, or if they don't want to take it, it may be possible to enroll in a study group using an alternative medication at a local teaching hospital. The decision will vary from woman to woman, but the important thing is not to be coerced into anything, but to make the decision from a position of informed choice.

The newest rationale for ET—to minimize the risk of cardiovascular disease—complicates matters even more. Although it is true that women are much more likely to die of heart disease than of breast cancer (currently 30 percent of women die of some form of CVD as compared with 4 percent of women who die of breast cancer), the advantages of ET are just not that clear-cut.

There is no question that "natural" estrogens in oral tablets maintain or increase blood levels of HDLs (the "good" lipids in the blood), but they also increase triglyceride levels. Many studies have found that high levels of total cholesterol and of the "bad" LDLs substantially increase the risks of heart attack but *only when triglyceride levels were also high.* It is suspected that triglycerides make the blood more likely to clot, which starts most heart attacks. It may well be that it is not only low HDLs and high LDLs that contribute to increased CVD risk, but that high triglycerides are an important and neglected part of the equation. (See also chapters 6 and 8.)

Women who have a family history of heart attack, or stroke, or who suffer from a chronic heart condition, may decide to take their doctor's recommendation and use ET, in the hope that current studies will validate this choice. But many healthy women recognize that there are other preventive strategies to reduce the risks of CVD and actually find the prospect of heart disease less frightening than the prospect of breast cancer. After all, we have to die of *something*, and what if we manage to avoid heart disease and then develop breast cancer at age eighty?

The whole question of estrogen use is highly complex, and there are no simple answers. Given the long latency period of breast cancer, it is hard to know just what was happening in a woman's body fifteen or twenty years ago, which results in a diagnosis of cancer today. Because types and doses of hormones have changed so much over the last few decades, it is impossible to go back and trace their possible effects. But even when we *do* have more definitive information, the decision about whether to seek or to accept hormone therapy has to be an individual one, based on the quality of life of one individual woman, and taking into account the many unknowns that still plague us.

REFERENCES AND RESOURCES

DeFazio, J. and L. Speroff. "Estrogen Replacement Therapy: Current thinking and practice," *Geriatrics*, *40*(11), November 1985.

Dejanikus, T. "Major drug manufacturer funds osteoporosis public education campaign," *The National Women's Health Network News*, May/June 1985.

Jensen, J., C. Christiansen, and P. Rodbro. "Cigarette smoking, serum estrogens and bone loss during hormone replacement therapy early after menopause," *New Engl. J. Med.*, *313*(16) October 17, 1985.

Kennedy D. L. et al. "Noncontraceptive estrogens and progestins: use patterns over time," *Obs. & Gyn.*, *65*(3), 441–446, 1985.

Leff, M., ed. "Do triglyceride measurements mean anything?" *Consumer Reports on Health*, *4*(8):59–60, August 1992.

Lindsay, R. "How calcium and estrogen combine to prevent osteoporosis," *Contemp. Obs. & Gyn.*:108–119, April 1986.

Lucisano, A. et al. "Ovarian and peripheral androgen and estrogen levels in post-menopausal women: correlations with ovarian histology," *Maturitas*, *8*, 1986.

Reed, M. J. et al. "Estrogen production and metabolism in peri-menopausal women," *Maturitas*, *8*, 1986.

Schiff, I. "Estrogen replacement at menopause," *Harvard Medical School Health Letter*, *12*(1), November 1986.

Shapiro, S. et al. "Risk of localized and widespread endometrial cancer in relation to recent and discontinued use of conjugated estrogens," *New Engl. J. Med.*, *313*(916), October 17, 1985.

Sturtridge, W. C. "Osteoporosis: Its assessment, investigation, treatment and prevention," *Geriatric Med.*, *1*, October 1985.

6

Increased Health Risks at Menopause: Osteoporosis, Heart Disease, Breast Cancer

For many of us, menopause comes as a shock. We are forced to become aware of what we take for granted—our bodies and our health. Because our bodies no longer respond, perform, acquiesce in the ways that they once did, we are forced to recognize our age and our mortality. Although some women find this difficult to accept, it does have its compensations.

Menopause reminds us to take stock of our health and to initiate steps to withstand the threats to good health that increase with age. It gives us the chance to decide whether we will be easy targets for diseases of old age or if we are willing to make an effort to stay healthy—not only for our own benefit, but for the benefit of those who would have to take care of us.

The word *osteoporosis*, which means porous bone, was first named by a German pathologist in 1930. Although extensive studies were done on postmenopausal osteoporosis throughout the 1940s and 1950s, it did not reach the popular press or stir up public concern until the 1980s. Osteoporosis is not a disease; it is the end result of many processes that

112

lead to a state where bone mass is less than the needs of body mass. Bone may appear normal but, on close inspection, is found to be riddled with holes, somewhat like a dry sponge. The bones of the forearm (near the wrist) and the thigh (at the hip) may become dangerously fragile, whereas bones in the spine threaten to collapse from the effort of holding up the body.

Heart-related medical conditions—hardening of the arteries, high blood pressure, heart disease, or stroke—account for more than half of the disabling health problems on this continent. Before age sixty, twice as many men are affected; after age sixty, women are as vulnerable as men. Menopause does not, of course, *cause* heart disease, but after age fifty-five, women are more likely to have high blood pressure (hypertension) than men. Any book about menopause must include the bad news: Menopause brings with it the increased risk of heart disease, particularly for those who experience surgical menopause. Once a woman has had one heart attack, her chances of experiencing a second are greater than a man's. And women are less likely to survive heart surgery. (See page 131).

We may be only vaguely aware of the heightened risks of osteoporosis and of cardiovascular disease, but many of us know, in some small, secret place, that we are also moving into a high-risk category for breast cancer. In fact, 65 percent of new cases of breast cancer occur in women over fifty.

Osteoporosis

Bone is both the vital framework of the body and a storehouse for calcium and other minerals. Bone cells are constantly being formed, used, and sloughed off, much like what happens on the outer layer of skin. The outer layer of bone sheds cells into the bloodstream, and the cast-off cells are excreted. The vast majority of calcium in the body exists as bone or teeth, but there is a constant circulation of calcium in the bloodstream. It is the balance between the loss of bone cells *(resorption)* and the formation of new cells *(absorption)* that determines bone density and presumed durability of bone.

During the growing years—until the mid-thirties—the absorption of calcium into bone exceeds the resorption of calcium into the bloodstream, so bones get bigger and stronger. Although we inherit a tendency to strong or weak bones, the density of bone can also be affected by the amount of calcium in the diet and by the weight and activity of muscle pulling against it—the action involved in all movement. If there is a family tendency to dense, durable bone, and if this is complemented by good nutrition and exercise habits, a negative balance (i.e., losing bone faster than it is formed) can be tolerated for some years. Men are generally heavier and more muscular than women and, until very recently, this difference was accentuated by men's wider participation in sports. This is the major reason why most men in our society do not show evidence of osteoporosis until well into old age. Because the life expectancy of the male is considerably less than the female, the problem of osteoporosis is overwhelmingly a woman's health problem in this society. (Although there have been slight changes, the average life expectancy of a woman is about six or seven years more than that of a man.)

There are two different kinds of osteoporosis: primary and secondary. Primary osteoporosis develops as a consequence of natural aging *in both men and women.* Secondary osteoporosis simply means that the condition is brought on, or worsened, as a result of other problems—prolonged bed rest, glandular disorders (hypoglycemia, hypothyroidism, Cushing's syndrome, Addison's disease, or diabetes mellitus), bone marrow tumors, kidney dialysis, and/or as a side effect of medication. Some of these medications are oral corticosteroids (e.g., prednisone for asthma), anticonvulsants (Dilantin), diuretics containing furosemide, or antacid preparations containing aluminum. Prolonged use of thyroid medication (particularly if the dosage is not reduced appropriately as a woman ages) increases the likelihood of osteoporosis, as does use of psychotropic drugs (tranquilizers, antidepressants, or sleeping pills).

Whether primary or secondary, the osteoporotic woman is at risk for crush fractures of the lower and/or upper back (the latter more evident as "dowager's hump"), for wrist fractures ("old lady's" or Colles' fracture), and for hip fractures—not at menopause but later in life. The immobility and complications resulting from hip fractures are responsible for the deaths of 20 percent of older women, usually within four months of the accident.

Osteoporosis is more common in affluent, northern countries where bone density peaks in the fourth decade of life. Most women then start losing between .02 and .07 percent of bone each year. During the two to five years immediately following the last menstrual period, bone loss may accelerate to as much as 2 percent (as a result of lowered estrogen levels) after which bone loss slows to the rate more characteristic of premenopause.

Women who have had multiple pregnancies, who eat red meat infrequently, who do strenuous labor, and who are overweight (by American standards) are not likely to develop osteoporosis. These are characteristics of the majority of women throughout the world. Moreover, black women rarely suffer from osteoporosis because they inherit denser bones than do whites. Asians in America, however, are vulnerable presumably because they tend to be small-boned and slim and because they do not inherit dense bone structure. (Ironically, Asians in China and Japan appear not to be as susceptible to osteoporosis. We are not sure why.)

Surgical removal of the ovaries doubles the risk of osteoporosis. Because North America leads the world in numbers of hysterectomies performed and since many surgeons still routinely remove ovaries from any woman over age forty or forty-five, the high incidence of osteoporosis is probably due to unnecessary elective surgeries. Interestingly, this is not viewed as a problem in the medical literature!

In addition to accelerated bone loss as a result of gynecological surgery or as a side effect of certain medications, some women fit into the category of "fast loser." Not a great deal is known about why certain women are "fast losers," but a blood test measuring the amount of a substance called *osteocalcin*, a bone GLA-protein, (when coupled with standard tests) will successfully identify nine out of ten women at risk.

Estimates about the prevalence of osteoporosis vary enormously. It is commonly believed that one in four women going through natural menopause, and one in three women experiencing surgical menopause, will be at serious risk, but this risk may only arise if and when a woman reaches her ninetieth year. Moreover, estimates of risk do not discriminate between those affected by less serious consequences of osteoporosis (minor vertebral compression, forearm fractures) and those disabled by crush or hip fractures, or their aftermath.

The Osteoporosis Risk Profile shown on pages 118 to 121 will give you an idea of your individual risk factors. Use this profile to help decide if you should be taking steps to protect yourself.

The best way to prevent osteoporosis is to have strong bones. Heredity is one factor, but women with strong bones will have consumed lots of calcium (milk, cheese, dark green vegetables) during their early adult years, and engaged in regular exercise that put stress on the bones. Because bone is built as the result of the mechanical pull of the muscles, exercises that involve use of the whole body are best—walking, running, rope-jumping, and racket sports. At one time it was thought that swimming was not particularly beneficial for osteoporosis because of the water's buoyancy. Now it has been found that swimming does help, although it cannot offer the same degree of needed stress to the bone as does weight-bearing exercise. Weight- or resistance training is good for the bones. Bicycle riding will help the bones of the lower body, but may not strengthen the bones of the arms and shoulders. (A cyclist who plays the piano regularly may have an advantage!)

Diagnosis

Bone loss is intensified by consuming a lot of caffeine (in coffee, tea, or soft drinks) and phosphorus (primarily in red meat and cola drinks), by smoking, and by not doing regular weight-bearing exercise. In addition to calcium, your diet should include adequate amounts of vitamin D ("the sunshine vitamin"), and three minerals—magnesium, manganese, and boron.

Women with fair, transparent skin seem more vulnerable to osteoporosis; the decline in mineralized collagen (bone) is reflected in the absence of opaque collagen under the surface of the skin. This skin type is also characteristic of rheumatoid arthritis sufferers, but what link exists between this and osteoporosis is not yet established. (Osteoarthritis, a noninflammatory degenerative joint disease, seems to add to the risk of osteoporosis. Women who have had a hysterectomy are at greater risk for both osteoarthritis and osteoporosis.)

Periodontal disease, which involves changes in the bones that hold the teeth in place or in the gum surrounding that bone, *may* be a sign of osteoporosis. One clue may be greater loss of bone in the upper jaw, which contains more trabecular bone than the lower. (Cortical bone, which constitutes 80 percent of bone mass, is the hard and shiny kind that makes up the outer surface. The inner part is called *trabecular*, or *cancellous*, and this more porous type of bone is characteristic of the major portion of the vertebrae. Trabecular bone is more vulnerable to osteoporosis than is cortical bone.)

Since the calcium that circulates in the blood helps to monitor muscle contraction, one early indication of calcium deficiency may be knotting of the large muscles, particularly in

OSTEOPOROSIS RISK PROFILE

This chart is intended to help you assess the extent to which you are at risk for spontaneous fractures of the spine, hip, and wrist that occur in persons with postmenopausal osteoporosis. Listed below are a number of factors that affect your risk profile, including those that can affect through your lifestyle ("takens"), as well as those that are genetically determined ("givens"). Beside each factor, find the statement that best applies to you, note the number beside that statement, and write the number in the right-hand column.

Givens

Score

Age:

Female—under 35 1   Age 35–50.............3   Age 51–65 7   Over 65 12   _____

Male—under 51 1   Age 51–65............2   Age 66–80.........3   Over 80 4   _____

Heritage:

African-American.........1   Asian...........2   Mediterranean or
                                               Middle Eastern 3   Nordic or
                                                                              Anglo-Saxon..........5   _____

Complexion:

Dark..........1   Ruddy/Olive 2   Fair/Pale 5   _____

118

Heredity:

No known bone problems in family 1

Relative over 60 with bone disease 3

Parent with bone disease 4

Relative under 60 with bone disease 5

_____

Wrist Size:

Over 6¼" 1

6"–6¼" 2

5¾"–6" 3

Under 5¾" 4

_____

Height:

Over 5'8" 1

5'5"–5'8" 2

5'2"–5'5" 3

Under 5'2" 4

_____

Body Type:

Mesomorphic (high muscle, low fat) 1

Endomorphic (high fat, low muscle) 6

Ectomorphic (low fat, low muscle) 6

_____

Gynecological Status

Still menstruating or postmenopausal after age 50 ..1

Menopausal or postmenopausal aged 46–50 3

Early menopause* at age 45 or under 5

Surgical menopause* age 45 or under 7

_____

* Deduct 5 points if estrogen therapy was started within one year after surgery or early menopause, 3 points if started more than three years after surgery or early menopause.

Total of "Givens" _____

119

Takens

Exercise

Total body exercise 4 or more times weekly....0
Total body exercise 1 to 3 times weekly....3
Total body exercise at least 3 times monthly....6
Tend to avoid any physical activity....12

Eating Habits

*Calcium intake***

More than 2 servings of dairy products daily ...0
4 or more servings of low-fat dairy products daily ...3
2 servings or less of dairy products daily....6
Do not eat dairy products if at all possible....12

**Subtract 3 points if you take a daily calcium supplement that provides from 500 mg to 1500 mg of calcium.

Protein intake

Seafood and white meat of poultry only....0
Avoid red meat altogether....1
Meat 3 times weekly or less....3
Meat 4 times weekly or more....6

Drinking Habits

Caffeine intake

Avoid caffeine and tannin beverages....0
Decaffeinated drinks and/or tea only....2
3 cups or less of coffee or tea daily....3
4 cups or more of coffee daily....6

Alcohol intake

| Weekly average:
Less than 2 beers, 8 oz.
wine, or 3 oz. spirits ......0 | Weekly average:
2 to 4 beers, 8–16 oz. wine,
or 3–6 oz. spirits ....2 | Daily average:
Up to 2 beers or 8 oz. wine
or 3 oz. spirits...............4 | Daily average:
More than 4 beers or 16 oz.
wine or 6 oz. spirits ......8 |

Tobacco Use:

| Nonuser ....0 | Occasional cigarette, less
than 14 weekly...........2 | Daily smoker but less than
10 daily....................5 | 10 cigarettes or more
per day ....8 |

Total of "Takens" _____

Add "Givens" (from page 119) _____

Final Total _____

Assess your risk according to the following:
8 to 25 = Risk well below average
26 to 48 = Risk below average
49 to 59 = Risk generally average
60 to 82 = Moderate risk
83 to 100 = Considerable risk

Note that this chart is not intended to diagnose whether you are or will be osteoporotic. It is simply an indication of the extent to which you are similar to women who have been found to have osteoporosis. For an accurate diagnosis, it is necessary to have a bone scan.

Profile created by Diane Palmason for *Fitness Leader*, October 1984. Used with permission.

the calf. (Low levels of potassium may also cause this kind of cramping, which can often be relieved simply by adding potassium-rich foods such as bananas to the diet.)

Seventeen years ago, I had my uterus and ovaries removed. I was taking estrogen for six years after that but finally decided to give it up as I dislike the idea of long-term dependency on a drug. Lately, I've been experiencing unbearable muscle spasms in my legs. I started eating a banana a day in order to alleviate the cramps, with absolutely no results. My doctor is as stumped about this as I am. Even regular exercise has not helped.

A common symptom of more advanced osteoporosis (usually postmenopausal) is lower back pain, either as a muscle spasm or dull ache. If the pain persists for several weeks and then disappears, it may signal the crushing of a vertebra. When bones are fragile, the smallest exertion—a sneeze or a hug—can cause a fracture.

Loss of height, particularly in the upper body, may also be an indication of osteoporosis. Some loss of height occurs naturally as one ages, due primarily to the contraction of the hip flexor muscles. But measurements of upper torso size may be an indication of bone health.

Although all the diagnostic methods used are noninvasive, painless, and involve little discomfort, some are more effective than others. Routine X-rays show loss only when 20 to 30 percent of bone is affected, often too late to take preventive action. CAT scans (computerized axial tomography) are available in large medical centers but must be specifically adapted and made available for osteoporosis. This often occurs only when the condition is so advanced that confirmation of diagnosis is sought.

To have a CAT scan, the woman is placed on a cot that is slid into a metal cylinder. The body is bombarded with rays that provide a computer printout of bone density. The CAT scan, neutron activation analysis (which is even more rare), and absorptiometry all use radioactive materials but expose the patient to only a fraction of that used in standard X-rays.

Dual photon absorptiometers or DPAs (also called *densitometers)*—or the newer DEXA, or dual energy X-ray absorptiometer—which measure bone mass in the spine and arm and then calculate and display results on a computer screen, have been acquired by most teaching hospitals and are the most common form of diagnostic instrument. Unfortunately, many are used only for research. Single photon absorptiometers (SPAs) are half the price but measure only forearm bone, and thus have not been as useful.

More and more hospitals are making bone scans available to the general public, so your physician may be able to make arrangements for a bone scan if you are worried about the risk of osteoporosis. The printout generated by a scan will tell you the state of your bones relative to other women your age. If your bone density is in the adequate range, you may decide to continue exercising regularly while taking calcium and vitamin D. (In areas of the country that get little winter sun, vitamin D is important. Spinal bone mass can be improved by taking 500 IU of vitamin D daily.) If the bone mass is "borderline," you may wish to have another scan in 12 months. If the results put you into or near the "fracture zone," you may decide to take estrogen. Estrogen will not strengthen existing bone but will halt the accelerated loss that occurs in the years around the last menstrual period.

The most telling symptom of osteoporosis is, of course, the broken bone. Once one fracture occurs, there is a tendency for other bones to break: 95 percent of osteoporotic women have at least five more fractures in the ten years following the first.

Nonprescription Remedies

There is a great deal of controversy over the role of calcium, particularly calcium supplements, in the prevention of osteoporosis among women who are premenopausal (still menstruating regularly), perimenopausal (having erratic or skipped periods), or postmenopausal (last period at least twelve months before). Because calcium is a nutrient, not a drug, its effects are not immediately apparent. And calcium alone is *not* enough to reverse the bone loss which marks the five years following the last menstrual period. But its effectiveness in building bone during the premenopause, and in strengthening bone in the years following year five of postmenopause, have been convincingly documented.

Most women consume only about 500 to 600 mg of calcium in their daily diet, which is below the RDA (recommended dietary allowance) of 800 mg daily, and the RDA itself is probably inadequate. According to a consensus panel of the National Institutes of Health, women *not* on estrogen should aim for 1400 to 1500 mg daily; those on estrogen need about 1100 mg.

Dietary sources of calcium are shown on pages 126 and 127. To consume enough daily calcium, a woman must diligently drink a quart of skim milk daily, or maintain a high intake of canned salmon or sardines (including bones), plus green, leafy vegetables. If this is impossible on a regular basis, it may be advisable to include a calcium supplement.

Calcium supplements, tablets designed to supplement the calcium in your regular diet, may offer inadequate protection for women *at high risk for* osteoporosis. But calcium supplements, *in combination with regular exercise*, are helpful for the average woman.

These supplements are available in many forms; the most common are calcium carbonate, calcium gluconate, calcium lactate, and dibasic calcium phosphate. The newest form is calcium citrate maleate, which is available in calcium-fortified orange juice. If you read the labels, you will find that calcium carbonate is 40 percent elemental calcium, dibasic calcium phosphate is 31 percent, citrate maleate is 24 percent, while lactate contains only 13 percent elemental calcium, and calcium gluconate only 10 percent. *It is the amount of elemental calcium that is crucial.*

In other words, a 600 mg tablet of calcium carbonate provides 240 mg of calcium, whereas the same size tablet of calcium lactate provides only 79 mg of calcium. Calcium gluconate provides even less. The labels of any calcium product available in a drugstore will indicate just how much elemental calcium you are getting. If you divide the price of the bottle by the units of elemental calcium, you will have a guide to the cost of this particular supplement. What you are looking for is the most economical product to do the job.

Cheaper isn't always better, however. To make sure your calcium tablet will be properly absorbed, put it in 6 ounces of white vinegar and see how long it takes to dissolve. If it is still virtually in one piece after thirty minutes, it is not likely to be effectively absorbed in the stomach.

Some forms of calcium are tolerated better than others. Calcium is absorbed more effectively along with a dairy product (milk or yogurt) and, for maximum benefit, just before bedtime. More new bone tissue is laid down while you sleep. If you have a bad reaction—indigestion, bloat, flatulence, constipation—to a particular calcium supplement, don't give up on calcium entirely. Try another product until you find one that you can tolerate. Avoid products that include other nutrients, such as vitamins A or D. When evaluating a product, it's better to deal with one nutrient at a time.

Calcium supplementation without exercise is probably a waste of money, because the calcium is likely to be excreted. Again, exercise is the key to prevention:

Research on postmenopausal women comparing exercisers to sedentary controls have consistently found exercise to be beneficial to bone health as measured by calcium balance, bone mineral content and cortical diameter. Particularly encouraging is that exercise has been found, not only to prevent bone loss, but actually to increase bone mass. In Smith's study of women aged 69 to 95, sedentary controls lost an average of 3.29 percent of bone min-

CALCIUM-RICH

Amount	Food	Calcium
Dairy Products		
Cheese		
1 oz.	Cheddar cheese	204 mg
1 oz.	Colby	194 mg
1 cup	Creamed cottage	126 mg
1 cup	Dry curd cottage	46 mg
1 cup	2% Cottage	155 mg
1 cup	1% Cottage	138 mg
1 oz.	Cream	23 mg
1 oz.	Feta	140 mg
1 oz.	Gouda	198 mg
1 oz.	Monterey Jack	212 mg
1 oz.	Mozzarella	147 mg
1 oz.	Part-skim mozzarella	183 mg
1 oz.	Low-moisture part-skim mozzarella	207 mg
1 oz.	Provolone	214 mg
½ cup	Ricotta	257 mg
½ cup	Part-skim ricotta	336 mg
1 oz.	Swiss	272 mg
1 oz.	American processed	174 mg
Milk		
1 cup	Whole (3.25% fat)	291 mg
1 cup	Low-fat (2% fat)	297 mg
1 cup	Low-fat (1% fat)	300 mg
1 cup	Skim	302 mg

eral over 36 months while those in an exercise program increased bone mineral by 2.29 percent.

—L. R. Gannon, *Menstrual Disorders and Menopause*

You will need adequate vitamin D to utilize the calcium properly. If you don't get regular exposure to sunlight (15 minutes a day is all it takes) and don't drink milk (100 IU of

FOODS

Amount	Food	Calcium
Milk (cont.)		
1 cup	Goat's	345 mg
Other		
½ cup	Ice cream	90 mg
½ cup	Ice milk	115 mg
1 cup	Plain yogurt	274 mg
1 cup	Plain low-fat yogurt	415 mg
Seafood		
1 cup	Oysters	226 mg
7.5 oz.	Pink salmon	160 mg
3.75 oz.	Sardines	240 mg
1 cup	Shrimp	147 mg
Vegetables		
1 cup	Bok choy	116 mg
1 cup	Broccoli	140 mg
1 cup	Collards	357 mg
1 cup	Dandelion greens	147 mg
1 cup	Kale	206 mg
1 cup	Mustard greens	193 mg
1 cup	Turnip greens	267 mg
Other		
4 Tbsp.	Almonds	85 mg
2 Tbsp.	Blackstrap molasses	280 mg
4 Tbsp.	Tahini	270 mg
3.5 oz.	Tofu	128 mg

D in each cup), you may need supplements: 400 to 800 IU daily.

Magnesium, manganese, and boron are minerals that are also necessary to maintain bone strength. The RDA for magnesium is 280 mg, available from whole-grain breads and cereals, and fresh, green, leafy vegetables. Studies have suggested that low levels of manganese in the diet are related to

poor calcium absorption and that the diets of most menopausal women are chronically short of manganese. There are no
RDAs established for manganese or boron, but 2 to 5 mg of
manganese daily is considered adequate; this is available from
whole grains, nuts, fruits, and vegetables. Preliminary studies suggest that boron may be vital to bone health, partly by
influencing estrogen levels during postmenopause. A diet
that includes lots of noncitrus fruits (apples, pears, cherries,
grapes), green vegetables (cabbage, broccoli, beet greens),
nuts and legumes (dried peas and beans, lentils) will provide
the necessary 2 mg to 6 mg.

Prescription Remedies

If your physical makeup and family history strongly pre-
dispose you to osteoporosis or if you have had a bone scan
and are perilously near the "fracture zone," you may want to
consider taking estrogen to halt further bone loss (although
you must *continue* to take estrogen to enjoy this benefit).
The most common prescription to prevent bone loss is one
.625 mg tablet of Premarin daily although the Estraderm
patch at 50 mcg offers equivalent protection. There is also
evidence that a reduced dose of Premarin (.3 mg) *with daily
exercise* may be as effective as .625 mg. Note, however, that
estrogen cannot build new bone in the absence of exercise.

Once a woman is five years postmenopausal, the period of
greatest bone loss is past. This is valuable information, because estrogen is often prescribed as if it works equally well
for all women, and as if all women were equally in need of it.

Research is underway to evaluate the bone-building potential of such medications as etidronate disodium (Didronel), medroxyprogesterone (Provera), and salmon calcitonin
(Salcatonin). Calcitonin is a hormone produced by the thyroid. It influences the level of calcium in the blood. Sodium
fluoride has received a lot of press in the last few years: it
definitely builds new bone, but the bone is structurally dif-

ferent from normal bone, and it's not yet known whether it can withstand the same kinds of stresses. In addition, sodium fluoride cannot be tolerated by everyone, and many women have had to stop taking it because of negative side effects.

Progesterone therapy (usually consisting of Provera, 10 mg daily, for ten days a month) is an alternative to estrogen for women who cannot take ET. Like sodium fluoride, progesterone appears to be most effective in rebuilding trabecular bone (which makes up most of the vertebrae). In one study, an 8 percent increase in bone density was achieved after one year of treatment.

A progestogen derivative with mild progestogenic, estrogenic, and androgenic effects has been developed (Org OD14, manufactured by Organon under the name *Livial*). This may have a significant bone-sparing effect without affecting the endometrium. It has been submitted for approval to the FDA.

Didronel is the newest star in the list of alternatives to estrogen. The most common regimen is two weeks of Didronel (400 mg daily) with thirteen weeks of no treatment; this fifteen-week cycle is then repeated ten times. After the first year or so of treatment, new bone growth is evident. Didronel has already been approved for the treatment of Paget's disease, which means it can legitimately be prescribed even though it is not FDA-approved for specific use in osteoporosis.

Calcitonin treatment, like estrogen, merely halts bone loss. In America, it is commonly administered by injection and is not only costly but often involves unpleasant side effects. In Europe, salmon calcitonin is available in a nasal spray to be inhaled once every other day. It has proved effective in treating bone loss in the spine, but is not yet approved for use in North America.

I am sixty-six years old and have been suffering from
osteoporosis for two years. Last winter, I broke my
hip in a fall and have since been extremely conscious

of my calcium and vitamin D intake. My doctor seems
to feel, however, that if I begin to take estrogen now,
the osteoporosis will decrease. Is this true?

Although estrogen *halts* bone loss, it cannot rectify the
effects of existing osteoporosis. But estrogen, together with
exercise, *can* rebuild lost bone; calcium is also effective, but
not to the same degree.

The promotion of ET to all women, to prevent osteoporosis, is based on projections of the costs of caring for older
women with broken hips. These projections are based on our
current situation, which is an aging population that has
never been encouraged to eat bone-building foods or to exercise regularly. Because most doctors have been trained to
look for medical solutions (drugs or surgery) to problems
presented by their patients, and because menopause has only
been fleetingly mentioned in medical school, most do not
think of adjustments in diet, or changes in exercise patterns,
as solutions. Younger women who are more aware of the
risks of osteoporosis—and of heart disease—are more likely
to get regular exercise and more likely to benefit from drug-
free remedies that may be less expensive and less risky.

Heart Health

Until recently, most studies dealing with heart disease focused on men. What was generally accepted to be true (in
terms of vulnerability to cardiovascular disease, or CVD)
was based on information about males. For instance, Type A
personalities—tense, ambitious overachievers—are considered more prone to CVD. More often than not, this means
male, middle-class management types. Among women, however, it is those earning low wages, with low status, who are
at greatest risk. These women are more likely to be blue-
collar, working class, in low-paying jobs.

Moreover, doctors are more likely to dismiss complaints of chest pain from women, judging it to be an emotional rather than a physical symptom. Men are also much more likely to be scheduled for angiography, a procedure involving injection of a dye that allows the blood vessels in the heart to be viewed on X-rays. And women who have bypass operations are less likely to survive, probably because by the time they are scheduled for surgery, they tend to be both older and more seriously ill than male patients.

Under the stewardship of Bernadine Healy, a cardiologist and the first woman director of the National Institutes of Health (NIH), women's susceptibility to cardiovascular disease, and the quality of medical treatment given to women, are undergoing new and very welcome scrutiny. We have a lot to learn.

The cardiovascular system is made up of four basic components: the pump (the heart), the pipes (the veins and arteries), the control system (the nerves that cause the heart to beat, valves that ensure the one-way flow of blood), and the material moving through the system (the blood). Problems may be caused by (1) clogging of the pump or pipes; (2) leaking or bursting of the pump or pipes; (3) breakdown in the control system; or (4) changes in blood as it moves through the system. Some problems result from a single cause, but most arise from a combination. The major culprit is the clogging of the pump or pipes.

The clogging starts when elements carried along in the blood coat, invade, and then accumulate on the inside of a blood vessel. The composition of the blood may be partly to blame, and the inner lining of the arteries may be roughened with wear, catching filaments as they flow by. But the particular pattern of the clogging and the locations are highly individual, and no one knows what causes a particular pattern. As the passage for the blood narrows, the heart must work harder to pump the blood into all the tissues. As the artery walls lose elasticity, they may weaken and balloon out. This is called an *aneurysm*. Should the aneurysm leak or burst, the consequences could be deadly.

In other cases, *thrombi* (blood clots) may hinder blood flow to the brain (cerebral thrombosis) or to the heart (coronary thrombosis). If the thrombus is swept along to another site to block circulation of the blood, it is an *embolism*. A *pulmonary embolism* occurs in the lungs; a *cerebral embolism* occurs in the brain.

When artery walls thicken and lose flexibility, the condition is known as *arteriosclerosis*. When the clogging is caused by deposits of certain kinds of fat *(atheromas)*, the condition is known as *atherosclerosis*. In order to force blood past these obstructions in the arteries, the heart must work harder which causes the pressure of the blood in the arteries to rise. This results in high blood pressure or *hypertension*.

Hypertension

A blood pressure reading is a routine part of every medical checkup. Blood pressure is charted according to the force of the heart pumping (the systole) over the force of the heart at rest (the diastole). Although the reading varies depending on amount of physical exertion, time of day, and emotional state, a consistent and acceptable reading is anything between 100 and 135 for the first number and between 50 and 85 for the second. A reading of 140 over 90 (written as 140/90) is considered borderline. The diastolic reading seems to be more important when predicting trouble.

Some women react to estrogen therapy with a sudden increase in blood pressure, which is why doctors recommend that women on estrogens have their blood pressure checked every six months.

Hypertension is known as the silent killer because you may have it and never know it. A person with high blood pressure is three times more likely to have a heart attack, eight times more likely to have a stroke, and five times more likely to experience heart failure. Hypertension may also lead to eye problems or kidney failure.

It was once thought that blood pressure naturally got higher as one aged. Now it is known that blood pressure can be kept at a healthy level through diet, exercise, reduced salt intake, by not smoking, by careful weight watching, and by adequate calcium in the diet.

> I am a woman of fifty-three who has been experiencing menopausal problems for five years. I was always a workaholic, smoked a lot, and generally ignored my health. I refused to let menopause slow me down although my blood pressure was high and I suffered from insomnia. Two years ago, I had a heart attack. I've now changed my lifestyle completely: I've stopped smoking, I eat better, and exercise regularly. My blood pressure is back to normal—thank God!—and I feel a hundred percent better.

When blood pressure rises, a doctor has the option of prescribing medication (usually a diuretic) or enlisting patient cooperation to change bad habits. Diuretics promote the excretion of fluids, including salt, but use of diuretics also causes frequent urination and loss of vital potassium. Strict antihypertensive drugs (and there are many of these) often involve even more side effects. One widely-used drug, reserpine, has been found to increase the risk of breast cancer; others lead to restless sleep and frequent awakenings. In addition, the benefits of hypertensive medication can be canceled by the interactive effects of other medications—oral contraceptives, appetite depressants, or nonsteroidal antiinflammatory drugs (NSAIDs) prescribed for arthritis.

More and more doctors recognize that a nondrug approach to controlling blood pressure may be as effective as medication, or more so. As much as one-third of the population is known to be sodium sensitive; for these people, a sharp reduction in salt intake may stabilize borderline blood pressure, which may then be treated with commonsense precautions—no smoking, more exercise, and a healthier diet.

Stroke

Leaking or clogging in the brain may lead to a major stroke (cerebrovascular accident, or CVA) or, if the leaking is intermittent and minor, to a transient ischemic attack (TIA). *Ischemic* simply means that the tissues are being starved of oxygen. If blood cannot reach brain cells, the starved cells will die. And, although some experts suspect that brain cells *may* have the capacity to regenerate, they don't know how to promote this regeneration. The damaged cells may never be reactivated; if many cells are affected, the result may be paralysis, loss of speech, or other deficits, depending on the part of the brain. Recovery is slow because new nerve pathways must be forged and old skills painfully relearned. If only a few brain cells are affected, the effects are more subtle— tingling in the extremities, momentary dizziness or weakness, etc. TIAs may be shrugged off as temporary inconveniences, but the cumulative effect of a series of TIAs may cause loss of brain function and even senility. At the end of a series of transient ischemic attacks, the patient's behavior may be similar to that of a person suffering from Alzheimer's disease.

Heart Attack

If leaking or clogging occurs in the coronary arteries, the diagnosis is *coronary heart disease* (CHD), or *ischemic heart disease* (IHD). The pain resulting from the heart's loss of its own blood supply is called *angina pectoris*. The usual progression is atherosclerosis of the coronary arteries, followed by ischemic heart disease (which makes itself known by the pain of angina), and finally a heart attack. The section of the heart fed by the clogged artery cannot function for more than five minutes without an adequate blood supply. When heart muscle is damaged, *myocardial infarction* occurs.

There are, of course, many other problems resulting from the leaking, clogging, and bursting of the heart and blood vessels. Some conditions are the result of birth defects; some result from scarring caused by a disease such as rheumatic fever; some are caused by bacterial infection or by conditions that affect specific parts of the heart or arteries.

Arrhythmia

Any disturbance to the natural rhythm of the heartbeat is arrhythmia, which is caused by a malfunction of the control system. The natural pacemaker of the heart functions inside the atrium, or upper chamber of the heart, and governs the regularity of the beat. *Tachycardia* is a condition in which the heart begins to beat too fast (at about 180 beats per minute). If the heart speeds up even more, it may flutter at around 250 beats per minute, or flatten out completely during *fibrillation.*

A less dramatic but more common complaint during menopause is paroxysmal atrial tachycardia, which does *not* lead to flutter or fibrillation and may occur in otherwise normal, healthy persons. Occasionally it may be caused by migraine activity (see chapter 2). Tachycardia is very different from the more common palpitations, which is merely an unpleasant awareness of the heart beating, and which is often felt at times of anxiety or panic.

If you experience episodes of tachycardia, you will be referred to a cardiologist to rule out rapid heart rate caused by the lower chamber of the heart, a more serious condition.

Medication is often routinely administered to alleviate arrhythmia, but recent studies indicate that skipped beats, or a temporarily "racing heart," rarely have any connection with heart disease. In fact, some studies suggest that the medication may cause more problems and that most people with heartbeat irregularities can expect to live as long and as healthily as anyone else.

The valves of the heart, arteries, and veins are a major part of the cardiovascular control system, because they ensure that the blood moves in the desired direction. Malfunction of the heart valves is not uncommon. When the mitral valve doesn't close properly after each beat, this can be heard through the stethoscope. In fact, prolapse of the mitral valve (Barlow's syndrome) is said to affect 15 percent of women over the age of thirty. There may be minor chest pain, some palpitations, and some shortness of breath after exertion. Echocardiography (a painless procedure that bounces sound waves into the chest cavity) can confirm the diagnosis of this syndrome, with relatively little risk. The greatest concern about mitral valve prolapse is the risk of heart infection, which can follow from standard dental procedures. Women with mitral valve prolapse are advised to keep a prescription for antibiotics on hand and to start ten days of treatment prior to any dental work (including teeth cleaning).

For the past year, I have suffered from severe heart palpitations and a very fast heartbeat. Cardiologists cannot find anything apart from a prolapse of the mitral valve, which apparently is of no concern. I have a spine full of arthritis, which causes pains in my neck, shoulders, and arms, and which some days is just about more than I can bear. This all hit me within a year after a lifetime of being just fine. I'm only forty-three and when I mention to doctors that perhaps I could be starting my change of life, they laugh at me. They think I'm too young for that. I get dizzy spells and tire very easily. I have had all the tests to be had and everything appears normal. I'm on beta-blockers to slow my heart down and I have side effects from this medication. So right now I feel like I have nowhere to turn. I know that I'm feeling like hell but the doctors apparently cannot or will not do anything for me.

Varicose Veins

The venous valves, particularly those below the waist, are responsible for varicose veins, which may occur quite aside from any conditions affecting the arteries. One can have varicose veins without any worry about arteriosclerosis, or clogged arteries. Varicose veins are estimated to affect at least 20 percent of women and perhaps 8 percent of men, and they seem to run in families. They may show up as a visible network of enlarged veins in the legs, as a painful ache from the veins deep inside the legs, or as hemorrhoids. They may be aggravated by pregnancy, when veins swell to accommodate the enormous increase in circulating blood.

Although varicose veins are not attractive, they are rarely life-threatening. Superficial veins may require elastic stockings (either heavy-duty elastic or the less noticeable support hose), which should be put on first thing in the morning before getting out of bed. Restrictive garments, such as girdles, knee-high stockings, tight shoes, or boots, and long periods of sitting or standing (especially if overweight) will make them worse. When sitting, the legs should be elevated as much as possible. A diet high in fiber and in vitamin C has been found to be beneficial. The superficial spiderweb-type marks that often accompany varicose veins may be treated with injections of saline solution, which often causes them to disappear. Ask your family physician for the name of a varicose vein specialist or sclerotherapist. Relatively painless minor surgery may be required for bulging surface veins, which can be "stripped," forcing the blood to circulate through deeper veins. The major risk with varicose veins is the possibility of blood clots (thrombi) or phlebitis, inflammation in the deeper veins.

Phlebitis

Although thrombophlebitis also involves veins, it is more serious and indicates the presence of both blood clots and inflammation. The presence of varicose veins increases the risk of phlebitis, as does taking the contraceptive pill. Deep-vein phlebitis is more difficult to treat. The inflammation (which causes a dull ache and/or swelling) may signal the presence of a clot (the thrombus) that must be dissolved using anticoagulants, which produce severe side effects in about 5 percent of patients. If the clot is not dissolved, it may loosen and move through the system to become a life-threatening embolism. Symptoms of an embolism may include chest pains or shortness of breath.

Blood clots may form after a blow to the legs, or a fall, or when blood flow is slowed down due to immobility, such as during illness or after surgery. Phlebitis is not common and is frequently misdiagnosed, but newer diagnostic tools (such as impedance plethysmography) are increasing medical expertise. Women prone to phlebitis are advised to exercise regularly and to give up smoking. Bedridden patients should be carefully monitored and, where necessary, low-dose anticoagulants used to increase blood flow.

Risk Factors for Cardiovascular Disease

Most of the factors that lead to increased risk of CVD can be controlled. The exceptions are heredity, age, and sex.

HEREDITY. Certain individuals may inherit a tendency to blood chemistry conditions that put a strain on the heart, such as high cholesterol levels, or prolonged abnormally-high white blood cell count. Afro-American women have higher rates of both heart disease and hypertension than whites, despite the fact that their blood cholesterol levels are often lower. The tendency to obesity, to dark hair in and around the inner ear, or to a crease across the earlobe are also inherited, and each is an indication of increased risk of CVD. Conversely, some of us also inherit a tendency to high HDL (high density lipoprotein) levels, which serve to protect against heart disease, or to varicose veins, which pose a minor risk. With some detective work, most of us can discover our inherited tendencies and work to offset them.

AGE/SEX. Age increases the risk for all forms of cardiovascular diseases; moreover, *women who experience any kind of menopause before the age of forty-five, and particularly forty, are at greater risk.* Women generally enjoy greater protection from most cardiovascular problems (as compared with men) until the late fifties, but are more prone to hypertension. Although it has been assumed that it is high levels of estrogen that provide the extra margin of protection to premenopausal women, ET administered to men results in more heart attacks. It's possible that high levels of testosterone in the male make him vulnerable, and that the risk diminishes as testosterone levels fall with age.

DIET. A high-fat diet significantly increases the risks of CVD, and excessive salt consumption is a primary factor in hypertension. There is still disagreement about the possible effects of coffee, although filtered coffee is safer than boiled or percolated (unfiltered) coffee.

Cholesterol is an animal fat found in many kinds of food (oils, meats, and eggs), but it is also manufactured by our bodies. The human liver can produce all the cholesterol we need. Because cholesterol and other fats (called triglycerides) are not water-soluble, they must be bound to other molecules that act as "carriers" in order to circulate in the blood. The carrier molecules are called lipoproteins. Lipoproteins fit into four groups according to density: Low-density lipoproteins (LDLs), in combination with cholesterol, are responsible for the congestion of artery linings and are a potential cause of heart disease. They are the "bad" lipids. High triglyceride levels may also be dangerous for women over age fifty. High-density lipoproteins (HDLs), on the other hand, pick up stray bits of cholesterol and dispose of them, counteracting the dangerous effects of the LDL/cholesterol combination, and are the "good" lipids. Menstruating women tend to have higher levels of HDLs than do men, which is one reason why younger women enjoy prolonged protection from cardiovascular disease. The concern with diet is to extend this protection past the menopausal years, so that women will remain at a lower risk for heart disease as they age.

A more complete explanation of the function of lipoproteins and how to evaluate cholesterol and lipid levels can be found in chapter 8. However, most of what we know about the role of the various kinds of lipoproteins in relation to heart disease has been the result of large-scale studies done on men who benefit from both the lowering of LDLs and raising of HDLs. Women's blood chemistry is different, and it is the shift in HDLs that is crucial.

The most recent theory suggests that excess iron in the system can be correlated to the probability of heart attack. The argument is that menstruating women are not prone to heart disease because the monthly bleed excretes excess iron, which can be stored indefinitely in the body. Further research is required, but it's possible that iron-rich foods (e.g., organ meats and spinach) may be poor choices after menopause.

ALCOHOL. Low alcohol consumption is related to lower probability of heart disease, hypertension, osteoporosis, and breast cancer.

SMOKING. Inhaled nicotine constricts the peripheral blood vessels, increasing resistance and thus blood pressure. A smoker is six times more likely to develop hypertension, because nicotine interferes with the liver's ability to dispose of blood fats, allowing more cholesterol and triglycerides to circulate and to clog up the system. At the same time, carbon monoxide in the cigarette smoke permits cholesterol to invade the artery lining and acts to reduce the oxygen-carrying capacity of the red blood cells. The risk of heart attack is directly related to the number of cigarettes smoked. Women who smoke are advised not to take the oral contraceptive pill after the age of thirty-five (even with the newer low-dose pills) until more consistent data are available.

STRESS. Risk of heart disease is also affected by stress. There is "good stress" and "bad stress." Stress produces a rush of epinephrine (another word for adrenaline)—a chemical that increases heart rate, blood pressure, and blood flow to the extremities. Evolution has programmed us to react swiftly to stress with heightened alertness and unusual physical strength. This enables us to run from the threat that produced the stress. We experience "good stress" when we rise to the occasion in a well-matched game of tennis or flog ourselves to swim another ten laps. If the chemicals are not dissipated through physical exertion, however, they can have damaging effects on the body. If these stressful episodes occur too frequently, or if any part of the cardiovascular system is weakened or damaged, chronic hypertension may result.

Stress occurring in a situation of powerlessness may be even more harmful. There is an enormous difference between the stress generated by high-powered women who thrive in pressure-cooker situations, and the stress endured by those women exploited by others, whether in a dead-end job or a no-win relationship. It is women in the latter situations who run the greater risk of hypertension and heart disease.

WEIGHT. A weight gain of 20 to 25 percent over "ideal weight" is considered obesity and poses a significant risk. Women who are overweight appear to be at greater risk for CVD than are overweight men, particularly if the extra weight is carried on the abdomen. If the waistline disappears and a "pot" develops, this is a warning sign. How the weight is distributed may be more important than sheer poundage. A gain of 10 to 15 percent over ideal weight (which may protect against osteoporosis and hot flashes) may be acceptable, provided the difference between waist and hip measurements remains roughly the same (e.g., instead of 26"/36" a change to 30"/40".)

EXERCISE. One of the best predictors of heart disease is a sedentary lifestyle. During exercise, most of the energy requirements for the muscles are provided by the blood. In order to provide increased oxygen during exercise, more blood pounds through the system as the heart rate speeds up, the rate of perspiration increases, and a larger amount of oxygen is extracted from the bloodstream by the organs and tissues. If the activity level is maintained, the arteries open up to increase the blood flow to working muscles. Exercise thus promotes the elasticity of the arteries, enhances blood flow, raises the level of HDLs in the blood, and reduces the probability of substantial weight gain. Regular aerobic exercise that sustains the heart rate at an optimum level for at least twenty minutes is one of the best ways to prevent cardiovascular problems. Chapter 8 provides a way of figuring out for yourself if you are getting sufficient, regular aerobic activity.

DIABETES: Women with diabetes are six times more likely to develop heart disease, as compared to male diabetics who incur double the risk.

We are handicapped by the limited information available about *women's* (as opposed to men's) heart disease: there appear to be significant differences not only in the development and symptoms of some kinds of cardiovascular disease, but also in the effects of certain treatments. Some women continue to produce ovarian hormones for many years after the last menstrual period; it is not known what effect this has on the risks of heart disease. Nor do we know what, if any, relationship exists among women who experience migraine, or severe varicose veins, or intense hot flashes, or palpitations associated with menopause. The current promotion of ET to protect women against CVD has obscured the fact that only very particular forms of ET have been found to be protective, and that this protection may reduce the risk of heart attack but not of stroke. We need much more information about women's individual risks.

Nevertheless, some women know they are at increased risk for CVD. Women who are dealing with known risk factors are anxious to see the results of current studies that may well establish the advantages of ET as a way of reducing certain risks. The most promising choice appears to be natural oral estrogens (e.g., Premarin at .625 mg), which have been demonstrated to increase HDL levels and protect against coronary heart disease.

Furthermore, even though we have known for some time that women who undergo artifical menopause continue to experience higher-than-normal risks of heart disease, there is no evidence of any concerted effort by the medical profession to reduce the unacceptably high rates of elective surgery. Until we have more accurate information, we are again faced with a situation where millions of women may be induced to take estrogen unnecessarily.

This might be acceptable if there were no negative long-term effects of estrogen therapy. But there is every indication that breast cancer rates will increase as a result of massive use of estrogen to protect women against heart disease.

The association of estrogen use and breast cancer remains speculative, but there is evidence that long-term use (for 10 years or more) can increase risk. . . . The cancer risk posed by progestins remains speculative as well; their effect on the breast in particular is a matter of controversy and has not been the subject of adequate investigation.

—OTA, *The Menopause, Hormone Therapy and Women's Health*, 1992:40

What to Do

In addition to maximizing heart health by cutting down on dietary fats, vitamin C has been reported to lower total cholesterol levels. Vitamin E is reputed to decrease blood coagulation, which could be helpful in preventing strokes. High fiber intake is important, because fiber binds with cholesterol (in bile acids) to move it out of the system. High calcium intake improves HDL levels and, together with exercise and vitamin D, also protects against osteoporosis. (Increasing milk consumption has been demonstrated to decrease blood pressure.)

Following up on studies of men who decreased the risk of stroke by consuming aspirin, it has now been decreed that women, too, can benefit. One low-dose aspirin, or as little as 30 mg daily, appears to reduce the threat of stroke. Coated tablets are available for those who find aspirin upsetting to the stomach.

Because these and other means of preventing heart disease, such as not smoking, healthy low-fat diets, exercise, and weight control have not been fully evaluated, we have no idea whether nonmedical preventive strategies might be as effective as estrogen supplementation in promoting a healthy old age. We *do* know that older women who exercise regularly and who maintain high HDL levels through the postmenopausal years have hearts and arteries characteristic of much younger women. More and more, we are recognizing that exercise may be the answer to a host of midlife health problems.

Breast Health

Five out of ten women see their doctors, at some point in their lives, about lumps, pain, swelling, or tenderness of the breasts. Pathologists have discovered that nine out of ten show some evidence of the kinds of cellular changes that we know as *fibrocystic breast disease*. But if nine out of ten women complain of lumpy breasts at some time or other, it must not be a *disease* at all, just part of being a woman. The fear of breast cancer can be alleviated to some degree when we recognize that lumps in the breast are normal, and that there are many different kinds of lumps. (Note that susceptibility to recurring fibrocystic breast lumps, when coupled with undiagnosed digestive difficulties, may be an early warning of ovarian cancer.)

Breasts are very individual parts of the body and there are great variations in size and shape. The left breast is often larger than the right; the nipple may or may not be inverted, large or small; the surrounding area (the areola) may be pale or dark, large or small. The internal structure is similar, however, made up of milk glands, forming lobes, which converge on the nipple through a series of ducts. Fibrous bands hold the lobes apart and attach the breasts to the chest wall. The supporting fibers are responsible for the "lift," which is affected by body weight, breast size, pregnancy, and breast feeding. Age brings about a thinning out of the fibers, with fatty tissue often filling up the spaces created.

Benign Breast Conditions

Although we tend to think of cancer whenever we notice anything unusual about our breasts, noncancerous breast conditions are much more common. Benign breast conditions may involve changes in the fibrous tissue, changes in the cells of the milk ducts, or the formation of cysts. The most common is the formation of cysts (chronic mastitis), which

Structure of the Breast

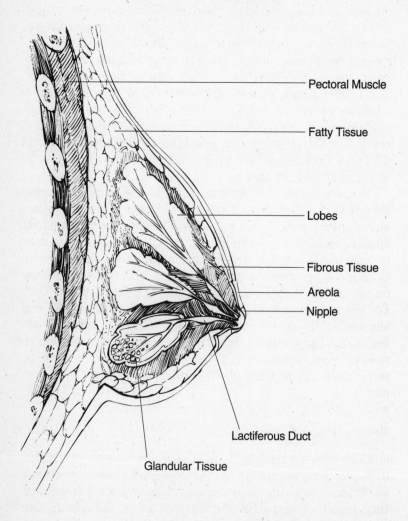

Pectoral Muscle

Fatty Tissue

Lobes

Fibrous Tissue

Areola

Nipple

Lactiferous Duct

Glandular Tissue

affects approximately 30 percent of women and tends
to be most bothersome between the ages of thirty and
forty.

> At the age of thirty-eight, I discovered lumps in my breast.
> Convinced I had cancer, I rushed to my doctor and
> was given no reason to believe otherwise. My doctor
> suggested that the lumps were probably cancerous and
> made an appointment for a mammogram and biopsy. As
> it turned out, it was cystic mastitis. The cysts were
> drained and I am grateful that it wasn't worse. I've
> learned to do routine breast self-examination (BSE) and
> I feel the importance of this cannot be stressed enough.
> Please pass this on.

It is not known why breast cysts form, but some relationship apparently exists between fibrous tissue, diet, and stim-
ulation by cyclical hormones. Before menopause, fluctuations
in estrogen tend to produce larger, more tender cysts prior
to menstruation, with changes in size and sensation following
the menstrual period. Generally cysts form hard, round
nodes that can be moved easily and that are filled with fluid.
There may be many small ones, a few medium-sized, or even
one large one. When they are too large and painful, they may
be aspirated (drained) with a fine needle. A darkish fluid—
yellow, green, or brown—is withdrawn and sent for routine
analysis. Cysts are rarely cancerous: the rare cancerous cyst
may have more to do with the cyst lining, which is smooth
when benign and irregular when malignant. Cysts often disappear spontaneously after menopause.

Methylxamine (found in coffee, tea, cola drinks, and chocolate) seems to aggravate formation of breast cysts. Nicotine
may also be a factor, because smokers seem to be more prone
to cysts. Low-fat diets have helped some women to reduce
the incidence and discomfort. Evening primrose oil has been
used by some women with promising results. Increased levels of vitamin A, vitamin B$_6$ (50 mg daily), and vitamin E

(800 IU daily in four doses of 200 IU), have also been used with excellent results. (For more information about vitamin E and some precautions about its use, see page 39.)

Changes in the fibrous tissue of the breasts can lead to a number of conditions. If a rubbery, painless tumor forms, this is a fibroadenoma. These tumors, which usually occur before age thirty-five, are not influenced by the menstrual cycle and move easily under the skin; they can usually be felt in the part of the breast closest to the armpit. A rare form of this condition may occur during menopause: giant fibroadenoma, also known as *cystosarcoma phyllodes* or *giant myxoma*. (I include all these terms just in case your doctor likes to bamboozle you with big words!) In the case of giant fibroadenoma, the lump grows rapidly to a large size and must be surgically removed.

Another rare condition that may also affect menopausal women is *fibrosis* (not to be confused with fibrositis), or *fibrous dysplasia*. This consists of a firm, painless mass with no defined edges, making it difficult to feel where normal tissue stops and abnormal tissue starts. Most of these fibrous tissue abnormalities are benign.

Breast cancer is much more likely to stem from changes in the milk ducts although, even here, very few conditions are "precancerous." Adenosis (which means abnormal growth) is a form of breast lump that may occur inside the milk duct. A lump under the nipple or areola may be caused by intraductal papillomas, which are wartlike growths that may produce a discharge from the nipple. An inflammation of the milk ducts, which is more common among postmenopausal women, is duct ectasia and may also produce nipple discharge.

It is estimated that up to 10 percent of women experience nipple discharge at one time or another. Some women have a white discharge for months after a baby is weaned. Others may notice a clear, or yellow, or reddish-brown discharge either occurring spontaneously or when the nipple is squeezed. Any discharge should be investigated, even though it is not unusual.

There are some serious forms of duct ectasia—*plasma cell mastitis* or *comedomastitis*. Occasionally the wartlike growths under the nipple are diagnosed as *ductal papillomatosis* and require intensive care. *Duct hyperplasia* (also known as hyperplastic disease) is a rare overgrowth of the lining of the milk ducts and is treated as a potential malignancy.

In addition to the four kinds of benign lumps already described—chronic mastitis, fibroadenoma, adenosis, and intraductal papillomas—a lump in the breast could be a lipoma (a fatty growth that can occur anywhere in the body) or fat necrosis (a hard lump resulting from a blow to the breast). Of all these kinds, textures, and sizes of breast lumps, only 10 to 15 percent will be malignant.

Breast Self-examination (BSE)

Many women shy away from breast self-examination despite the massive promotional efforts of the American Cancer Society. Unfortunately, the emphasis on BSE has been to *find lumps* rather than to become more familiar with a healthy part of the body. Most of us are very familiar with our neck and throat. We feel the neck as we adjust jewelry or fix our hair. We notice small changes—a gland swelling under the jawline, an odd bump behind the ear, a small bump, perhaps a mole, which we can feel but which is out of sight in the mirror. We monitor the state of the neck regularly and quite unself-consciously. Why can't we bring this same attitude to breast examination?

The steps involved are neither difficult nor time-consuming. Looking carefully at oneself in the mirror is easy. But the problem, for many of us, is the actual palpation—searching with the tips of the fingers for anything unusual. It is difficult to find anything unusual if one is not accustomed to the *usual*.

Many women have learned to examine their breasts while in the shower or in the tub, where soapy fingers or shower

BREAST SELF-EXAMINATION:
A New Approach

All women over 20 should practice monthly breast self-examination (BSE). Regular and complete BSE can help you find changes in your breasts that occur between clinical breast examinations (by a health professional) and mammograms.

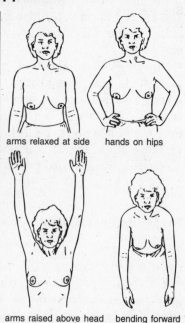

arms relaxed at side   hands on hips

Women should examine their breasts when they are least tender, usually seven days after the start of the menstrual period. Women who have entered menopause, are pregnant or breast feeding, and women who have silicone implants, should continue to examine their breasts once a month. Breast-feeding mothers should examine their breasts when all milk has been expressed.

If a woman discovers a lump or detects any changes, she should seek medical attention. Nine out of ten women will not develop breast cancer and most breast changes are not cancerous.

arms raised above head   bending forward

Remember the seven P's for a complete BSE: 1. Positions 2. Perimeter 3. Palpation 4. Pressure 5. Pattern 6. Practice and Feedback 7. Plan of Action.

1 POSITIONS
In each position look for changes in contour and shape of breasts, color and texture of the skin and nipple, and evidence of discharge from the nipples.

Palpation: Side lying and flat. Use your left hand to palpate the right breast, while holding your arm at a right angle to the rib cage, with the elbow bent. Repeat the procedure on the other side. The side-lying position allows a woman, especially one with large breasts, to most effectively examine the outer half of the breast. A woman with small breasts may need only the flat position.

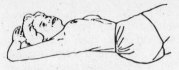

Side-lying position: Lie on the opposite side of the breast to be examined. Rotate the shoulder (on the same side as the breast to be examined) back to the flat surface.

Flat position: Lie flat on your back with a pillow or folded towel under the shoulder of the breast to be examined.

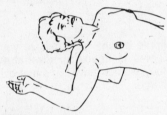

2 PERIMETER

The examination area is bounded by a line which extends down the middle of the armpit to just beneath the breast, continues across along the underside of the breast to the middle of the breastbone, then moves up to and along the collarbone and back to the middle of the armpit. Most breast cancers occur in the upper outer area of the breast *(see shaded area in illustration).*

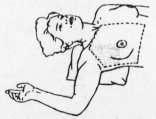

3 PALPATION WITH PADS OF THE FINGERS

Use the pads of three or four fingers to examine every inch of your breast tissue. Move your fingers in circles about the size of a dime. Do not lift your fingers from your breast between palpations. You can use powder or lotion to help your fingers glide from one spot to the next.

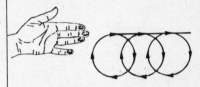

4 PRESSURE

Use varying levels of pressure for *each palpation,* from light to deep, to examine the full thickness of your breast tissue. Using pressure will not injure the breast.

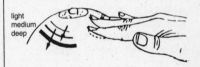

light
medium
deep

5 PATTERN OF SEARCH

Use one of the following search patterns to examine all of your breast tissue. Palpate carefully beneath the nipple. Any incision should also be carefully examined from end to end. Women who have had breast surgery should still examine the entire area and the incision.

Vertical strip: Start in the armpit, proceed downward to the lower boundary. Move a finger's width toward the middle and continue palpating upward until you reach the collarbone. Repeat this until you have covered all breast tissue. Make at least six strips before the nipple and four strips after the nipple. You may need between 10 and 16 strips.

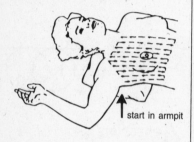

start in armpit

Wedge: Imagine your breast divided like the spokes of a wheel. Examine each separate segment, moving from the outside boundary toward the nipple. Slide fingers back to the boundary, move over a finger's width and repeat this procedure until you have covered all breast tissue. You may need between 10 and 16 segments.

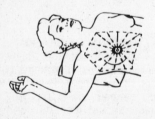

Circle: Imagine your breast as the face of a clock. Start at 12 o'clock

and palpate along the boundary of each circle until you return to your starting point. Then move down a finger's width and continue palpating in ever smaller circles until you reach the nipple. Depending on the size of your breast, you may need 8 to 10 circles.

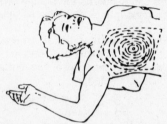

Nipple discharge: Squeeze your nipples to check for discharge. Many women have a normal discharge.

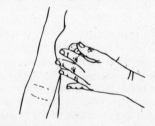

Axillary Examination: Examine the breast tissue that extends into your armpit while your arm is relaxed at your side.

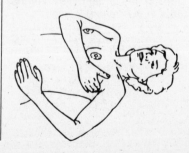

6 PRACTICE WITH FEED-BACK

It is important that you perform BSE while your instructor watches to be sure you are doing it correctly. Practice your skills under supervision until you feel comfortable and confident.

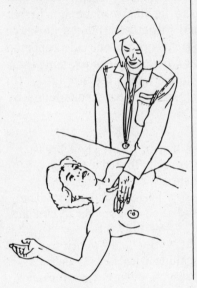

7 PLAN OF ACTION

Discuss the Cancer Society breast cancer detection guidelines with your health professional.

Schedule your clinical breast examination and mammogram as appropriate.

Do monthly BSE. Ask your health professional for feedback on your BSE skills.

Report any changes to your health care professional.

Reprinted with permission from the American Cancer Society, California Division, Inc.

gel allow for more comfortable manipulation of breast tissue. Baby oil also helps, so you might wish to ask your doctor to use it to make breast examination more comfortable for you. When we realize that the odds are very much in our favor— that we are likely to find everything normal or a harmless condition that can be easily treated—it is easier to stick to a resolution to examine the breasts once a month.

There are no records of the incidence of benign breast conditions noticed, treated, and forgotten. But we do know that 85 to 90 percent of breast cancers are initially reported by women doing BSE, and that women who *do* examine their breasts regularly are able to notice lumps the size of the tip of a ballpoint pen, lumps much smaller than those found by experienced doctors.

In January last year I had a biopsy on my right breast which showed a carcinomic growth. To make a long story short, the cancer had spread to my spine and the blood tests showed it was a hormone-fed cancer. The clinic recommended cobalt radiation treatments to irradiate the ovaries. Needless to say, I was fully into menopause literally overnight, with about twenty to thirty hot flushes daily. One thing I learned: If there is any visual change in your breasts—even if a lump cannot be found—get to a doctor immediately and keep going until you find a doctor who will listen to you. I had a dimple in my breast. I got worried when the doctor couldn't feel a lump. The dimple kept getting larger. Listen to your intuition because you know your body better than anyone else, including all doctors!

Diagnosis

Because of the increased risk of breast cancer in midlife, many physicians now routinely send their patients for a mammogram. The referral to the Radiology Department or a and, during a second operation to remove a quarter of my breast, lymph node involvement was found. I have presently had two bouts of chemotherapy with six to go. Four years ago, my sister (who is five years younger than me) had a mammogram, which was clear. She was experiencing menopausal problems and her doctor prescribed estrogen. When they discovered that I had breast cancer, she asked for another mammogram and, sure enough, she has it, too! She, like me, had a lumpectomy and is presently undergoing radiation therapy. Both our tumors were less than 1 cm and the prognosis is good, but I'm afraid I feel we would never have had these cancers if it weren't for estrogen. As soon as the cancer was diagnosed I was taken off estrogen and put on tamoxifen, an antiestrogen. I was told the other day that my tumor has estrogen receptors. It makes me sick to think that for four years I was feeding the thing. I should mention that my older sister has been on estrogen for about ten years and is fine. I guess not everyone is going to get cancer from taking estrogen, but I would not wish what I have been through on anyone. I think the risk is too great.

Some breast cancers are hormone-dependent, in which case treatment is directed toward reducing hormone levels in the body as quickly and as completely as possible. Other cancers do not react to hormones and still others appear to be a mixture of the two. There are contradictory reports about the long-term effects of oral contraceptives on breast cancer. Some say that long-term pill users are at decreased risk; some say the contrary. Synthetic estrogen in the form of diethylstilbestrol (DES)—once routinely administered to reduce the risk of miscarriage—is now known to be associated with levels of breast cancer at least 30 percent higher than normal in the women who were given it. ET is suspected to cause an increase in breast cysts and fibrous lumps, but we

clinic does *not* mean that anything unusual has been detected. If you have seen the doctor because of a lump, it may be biopsied in the doctor's office; if anything unusual shows up on the mammogram, you will be sent for a biopsy. Rather than becoming alarmed about incipient cancer, we should learn to accept mammograms and biopsies as routine procedures in the maintenance of good health. We don't panic about getting standard blood tests or chest X-rays, although each could just as easily point to some kind of abnormality. As we get older, it seems important to look at a biopsy in the same way—just one more standard test that helps to confirm our continuing good health.

There are a number of ways to examine breast tissue without breaking the skin. Thermography uses heat sensitivity to map areas where there is rapid cell growth (assumed to be tumors) and to contrast this with normal tissue. However, a mild inflammation may produce heat, so for this and other reasons, thermography has not been found to be consistently accurate. Transillumination (and a more recent offshoot of this, diaphanography) uses a bright light shining against the breast to show up darker masses of tissue. The accuracy of these methods depends on the density of the breast tissue. So far, they are useful only in conjunction with other methods. Ultrasound, which can differentiate fluid-filled cysts from solid masses, is less reliable after menopause, when the breast tissue changes (and when cysts tend to disappear anyway). Any or all of these methods may be used if the breast condition is judged to be benign and if the woman refuses mammography.

Menopausal women have breasts that are better suited to mammography than are the breasts of younger women. At midlife, breasts become less fibrous and more fatty, yielding the high contrasts needed for accurate diagnosis. Postmenopausal women on ET or CHT have denser breasts than women not receiving hormone therapy; increased density slightly diminishes the sensitivity of mammograms for early detection. Long-term effects of mammogram radiation may be worrisome to younger women but, by age fifty, we can afford to worry less; it is estimated that it would take at least thirty years for any radiation effects to show up. More attention is being paid to state-of-the-art machines. Currently, it is recommended that a baseline mammogram be done at age forty, followed by regular annual mammograms. If there is breast cancer in the immediate family, some experts recommend that examinations start at a younger age and be scheduled every six months.

When you call to schedule your mammogram, ask about the facilities: Is the equipment used solely for mammography? Is the radiation dose 0.4 rads or less? Are the technicians trained specifically in mammography and certified by the American Registry of Radiologic Technologists? Is the radiologist who reads the plates board-certified (American Board of Radiology or American Osteopathic Board of Radiology)? Does the radiologist read adequate numbers of mammograms (preferably several daily)?

The mammogram is usually conducted by a female technician in privacy and is a short and relatively painless procedure. Each breast is placed between two plates and pressure exerted to compress it as much as possible—once horizontally and once vertically. There are many rumors about the pain of mammography, but I have found that such complaints are not widespread. Women with larger than normal breasts are likely to find it uncomfortable, and the sensation of cold steel against warm flesh is not pleasant. However, the newer machines use warmer substances and some exert the final fractions of compression automatically as the technician steps into the booth or allow the woman herself to finish the compression. This means that the worst sensation of squeezing is very brief. If you do have the misfortune of running into an insensitive technician, be sure to complain to the person in charge.

Because postmenopausal women no longer have menstrual cycles to account for the size or tenderness of breast lumps, any lump will be treated with suspicion. In addition,

because the odds of breast cancer increase with age, doct are on the alert for any abnormality. If you report findir lump, your doctor may want to perform a quick, wide-ne biopsy in the office. This is done using a local anest (which freezes the area) and a second needle to draw sample of cells. Sometimes the procedure is done at an patient Clinic.

Breast Cancer

Despite the variety and frequency of benign breas tions, to most women the term breast health me avoidance of breast cancer. Because our cultur breasts primarily as symbols of femininity and sexu reason why we may be reluctant to examine them us harbor an irrational fear of breast cancer. We selves that we are not at risk, even though 70 to of new cancers are diagnosed in women who are n cific risk category. This is how fear gets in the w ble self-care.

If your mother or a sister has (or has had) br you are at higher than normal risk. If you have pregnant, or had your first child after age thirty breast feed, you are at slightly higher risk than you had an early menarche (first menstrual pe late menopause, the risk is increased. And final overweight and eat foods high in fats, your r Some of these risk factors cannot be changed, worth knowing about—if not for you, then for eration.

Some years ago I had my first mammogram clear. This was because my left breast incli a bit fibrocystic so nothing could be seen. there was something there, but in my righ couldn't feel it, though. It turned out to b

don't know enough about its effects in relation to breast cancer. (For more about this, see chapter 5.)

On rare occasions, a woman may notice that her nipple is itchy, red, and weeping. It may look and feel like a simple skin infection, but home remedies such as salves and lotions won't help. It's time to see a doctor. It could be Paget's disease, which is a rare form of cancer (not to be confused with Paget's disease of the bone).

Because breast cancer is probably two or three different diseases (one of which may affect only postmenopausal women), there are many different treatments. If you know women who have breast cancer, you may find the differences in their treatments confusing. This does not necessarily reflect different attitudes of their doctors, but rather different types of cancer.

If you *do* find a lump in your breast and it *does* turn out to be malignant, the prospects for full recovery are better than they've ever been. About 70 percent of early-stage breast cancers are cured by surgery; the balance will require radiation and/or surgery plus drug therapy. Cancers will recur in only about one-third of the remaining 30 percent. Because most surgeons prefer to perform a lumpectomy (which removes the lump and leaves the breast virtually intact) where possible, rather than the traditional but disfiguring removal of the breast (mastectomy), the odds of losing a breast, either with or without underlying muscle and/or underarm lymph nodes, have been markedly reduced. Whether lumpectomy or mastectomy, adjuvant (drug) therapy and/or radiation treatments are also frequently recommended.

When cancer is diagnosed, try to find a strong friend to lean on. Discuss your options. If your doctor insists that you have the procedure *he* or *she* recommends, be sure to get a second opinion. (See chapter 7 for details.) Not only should you insist on a second opinion, but you should also insist on time. Women have, too often, been wheeled into an operating room not knowing whether they would emerge whole or not. It is generally conceded that, even in extreme cases, women

should be permitted two separate procedures—first the biopsy and later, after advice and deliberation, a second operation. Most of all, women need support and friendship to resist
hasty decisions.

The incidence of *never-discovered cancer* in women over
the age of seventy (who have died of other causes) is nineteen times that of discovered (palpable) breast cancer. This
means that, for every woman who has a breast lump diagnosed as malignant, there are nineteen women whose breast
lumps never grow—lumps that appear but never get larger,
or disappear, or grow so slowly as never to be noticed. Experts believe that the seeds of potentially cancerous lumps
are with us from puberty onward, when the breasts first develop, but how our immune system acts to stop these lumps
from developing is still a mystery.

So breast cancer is probably not something that we "get,"
like a cold or the flu. Environmental factors—pollutants,
chemicals, diet, and even stress—may play a part. But the
seeds of breast cancer are already sown in each of us and are
as unpredictable and unexpected as all those other lumps—
whether cysts, adenomas, adenosis, lipoma, or fat necrosis.

The fear of breast cancer has led to the present-day trials
of tamoxifen (Nolvadex) using healthy women who are at
risk of—or more likely frightened about—breast cancer. (A
women of sixty with no known risk factors, aside from her
age, is considered to be at equal risk to a woman of thirty-
five with a strong family history of breast cancer. Remember,
too, that more than seven out of ten new cases of breast cancer occur in women with no known risk factors).

Tamoxifen is an antiestrogen that has proven successful
as adjuvant drug therapy for women who have been treated
for established breast cancer, reducing the risks of recurrence. Tamoxifen induces a pseudo-menopause (including hot
flashes, night sweats, and possibly nausea and depression) in
the short term; we still don't know much about long-term effects.

It strikes me as ironic that otherwise healthy women who are frightened of getting breast cancer should be asked to take a drug that will induce menopausal symptoms, while otherwise healthy women who experience menopausal complaints are being urged to take a drug that may increase their risks of breast cancer. *What* is going on?

REFERENCES AND RESOURCES

Albers, M. M. "Osteoporosis: A health care issue for women," *Health Care for Women Internatl.*, 11:11–19, 1990.

American Cancer Society, 19 West 56th St., New York, NY 10019 (212-586-8700).

Berkowitz, G. S. et al. "Estrogen replacement therapy and fibrocystic breast disease in postmenopausal women," *Amer. J. Epidem.*, 121(2), 1985.

Bush, T. L. and E. Barrett-Connor. "Noncontraceptive estrogen use and cardiovascular disease," *Epidemiologic Reviews*, Johns Hopkins U. School of Hygiene and Public Health, 7:80–104, 1985.

Cauley, J.A. et al. "The relationship of physical activity to high density lipoprotein cholesterol in postmenopausal women," *J. Chron. Disease*, 39(9):687–697, 1986.

Cobb, J. O. "New hope for old bones," *A Friend Indeed*, 8(2), May 1991.

Cobb, J. O. "Mammography and breast self-examination: We need both," *A Friend Indeed*, 8(6), November 1991.

Cobb, J. O. "The tamoxifen trials," *A Friend Indeed*, 9(5), October 1992.

Cobb, J. O. "Where the women are," in Lorrain, Plouffe, Ravnikar, Speroff and Watts, eds., *Comprehensive Management of Menopause*, NY: Springer-Verlag, 1993.

Colditz, G. A. et al. "Menopause and the risk of coronary heart disease in women," *New Engl. J. Med.*, 316(18), April 30, 1987.

Dawson-Hughes, B. et. al. "A controlled trial of the effect of calcium supplementation on bone density in postmenopausal women," *New Engl. J. Med.*, 323(13);878–883, 1990.

Dawson-Hughes, B., G. E. Dallal, E. A. Krall et al. "Effect of Vitamin D supplementation on wintertime and overall bone loss in healthy postmenopausal women," *Ann. Intern. Med.*, 155(7):505–512, 1991.

Geriatrics, 43(5):90, May 1988.

Hasselbring, B. "New and improved breast self-examination," *DES Action Voice*, #32, Spring 1987.

Heaney, R. "Estrogen-Calcium Interactions at the Menopause," Paper presented at the meetings of the North American Menopause Society, Cleveland, Ohio, September 1992.

High Blood Pressure Information Center 120/80, NIH, Bethesda, MD 20892 (301-496-1809).

Hreschyshyn, M. M. et al. "Effects of natural menopause, hysterectomy and oophorectomy on lumbar spine and femoral neck bone densities," *Obs. & Gyn.*, *72*(4) 1988.

Lapidus, L. et al. "Triglycerides—Main lipid risk factor for cardiovascular disease in women?" *Acta Med. Scand.*, *217*:481–489, 1985.

Lapidus, L. et al. "Concentrations of sex-hormone binding globulin and corticosteroid binding globulin in serum in relation to cardiovascular risk factors and to 12-year incidence of cardiovascular disease and overall mortality in postmenopausal women," *Clin. Chem.*, *32*(1):146–152, 1986.

Lapidus, L. "Ischemic heart disease, stroke and total mortality in women: Results from a prospective population study in Gothenburg, Sweden," *Acta Med. Scand. Suppl.*, *219*:1–42, 1986.

LaRosa, J. C. "Effect of estrogen replacement therapy on lipids: Implications for cardiovascular risk," *J. Reprod. Med.*, *30*(10), 1985.

Leff, M, ed. "Mammograms: Crucial but fallible," *Consumer Reports on Health*, *3*(12):89–91, December 1991.

Love, S. *Dr. Susan Love's Breast Book*. Reading, MA: Addison-Wesley, 1990.

Lubin, F. et al. "Overweight and changes in weight throughout adult life in breast cancer etiology," *Am. J. Epidem.*, *122*(4), 1985.

Melton, L. J. III. "Epidemiology of osteoporosis: Predicting who is at risk," in *Multidisciplinary Perspectives on the Menopause* (Annals N.Y. Acad. Sci., 592) 295-306, 1990.

Napoli, M. A. "New study questions breast cancer detection tests for young women but finds value to those over 50," *HealthFacts*, July 12 (98), 1987.

National Diabetes Information Clearinghouse, P.O. Box NDIC, Bethesda, MD 20892 (301-468-2162).

National Institute on Aging, U.S. Dept. of Health and Human Services. *The Healthy Heart Handbook for Women*, NIH Pub. #89–2720, Washington, DC: U.S. Government Printing Office, 1989.

National Institutes of Health, *What You Need to Know About Breast Cancer*. NIH Publication #91–1556. Washington, DC: U.S. Government Printing Office, 1991.

National Osteoporosis Foundation. *Osteoporosis: A Woman's Guide*. Washington, DC: The Natl. Osteo. Found. Publications, 1987.

Notelovitz, M. "Exercise and health maintenance in menopausal women," in *Multidisciplinary Perspectives on the Menopause* (Annals N.Y. Acad. Sci., 592):204–220, 1990.

Pick, R. "Atherosclerosis: The risk factors for women," *The Female Patient*, *2*:60–71, 1986.

Prince, R. L. et al. "Prevention of postmenopausal osteoporosis," *New Engl. J. Med., 325:*1189–1195, 1991.

Prior, J. C. et al. "Spinal bone loss and ovulatory disturbances," *New Engl. J. Med., 323:*1221–1227, 1990.

Richelson, L. S. et al. "Relative contributions of aging and estrogen deficiency to postmenopausal bone loss," *New Engl. J. Med., 311:*1273–1275, 1990.

Sartoris, D. J. et al. "Progress in radiology: Dual-energy radiographic absorptiometry for bone densitometry," in *Multidisciplinary Perspectives on the Menopause* (Annals N.Y. Acad. Sci., 592) 307–325, 1990.

Sherman, B., R. Wallace and J. Bean. "Estrogen use and breast cancer: Interaction with body mass," *Cancer, 51:*1527–1531, 1983.

Silfverstolpe, G. and N. Crona. "Hormonal replacement therapy—cardiovascular disease," *Acta Obstet. Gynecol. Scand. Suppl., 134:*93-95, 1986.

Stampfer, M. J., G. A. Colditz, W. C. Willett et al. "Postmenopausal estrogen therapy and cardiovascular disease—10-year follow-up from the Nurses' Health Study," *New Engl. J. Med., 325:*756–762, 1991.

Stomper, P. C., V. J. Van Voorhis, V. A. Ravnikar, J. E. Meyer. "Mammographic changes associated with postmenopausal hormone replacement therapy: A longitudinal study," *Radiology, 174*(2):487–490, 1990.

U.S. Congress, Office of Technology Assessment, *The Menopause, Hormone Therapy, and Women's Health,* OTA–BP–BA–88 (Washington, DC: U.S. Government Printing Office, May 1992).

Vandenbrouke, J. P., "Postmenopausal estrogen and cardioprotection," *Lancet, 337:*833–834, 1991.

Walsh, B. W., I. Schiff, B. Rosner et al. "Effects of postmenopausal estrogen replacement on the concentrations and metabolism of plasma lipoproteins," *New Engl. J. Med., 325:*1196–1204, 1991.

Watts, N. B. et al. "Intermittent cyclical etidronate treatment of postmenopausal osteoporosis," *New Engl. J. Med., 323:*73-79, 1990.

Wingo, P. A. et al. "The risk of breast cancer in postmenopausal women who have used ERT," *J. Amer. Med. Assoc., 257:*209–215, 1987.

7

Menopause Under the Knife: Common Surgical Procedures

Although none of the surgical procedures described in this chapter is unique to menopause, they are procedures that the menopausal woman should know about. This is particularly true of hysterectomy, which may bring on an earlier than normal menopause, and oophorectomy (or ovariectomy), which causes immediate and severe menopause. If surgery is recommended, such as for heavy or irregular bleeding, women may readily agree to an operation, because they're too frightened to explore other avenues. This may be one reason why such an unusually high number of operations are performed on women.

Deciding About Surgery

It is no surprise that surgery is more likely to be proposed by a surgeon than by another type of physician. Gynecologists are surgeons, and one of the strongest predictors of high rates of hysterectomy in a given area is the number of surgeons. In England, where fewer surgeons are trained as a proportion of all medical doctors, the rates for many standard surgical procedures are significantly lower. For instance, only 11 percent of English women have hysterectomies, as compared with 25 to 35 percent in the United States. In fact, it is the discrepancy between rates of surgery from one country to another, and from region to region within this country, which has led medical insurance companies to require a second opinion before agreeing to cover surgeons' fees. Those of us concerned with women's health recommend that you *always* get a second opinion. If you are contemplating major surgery, you may even want a third opinion.

To get a second opinion, you should consult a doctor whose opinion is likely to be independent from the first. This will involve finding a doctor with a different hospital affiliation, of a different age group, with offices in a different area. Find someone who is *not* part of the same "old boys' network." A good family physician or general practitioner is more likely to consider other options before recommending "the knife." No reputable surgeon will object to a second or third opinion and, if you feel you are being pressured into an operation, you should stand firm. The time you take to make decisions *before* surgery has a lot to do with your psychological well-being *after* surgery.

If you decide to go ahead with the surgery, you should have every confidence in the doctor who performs the operation. Sometimes it's possible to get valuable information by telephoning the operating room nurses who assist the surgeon. Make sure your potential surgeon is board certified by the American Board of Obstetricians and Gynecologists, and ask how many similar procedures this person has performed. You may also want to talk to some of his or her patients to find out if the doctor stays just as involved and concerned *after* the operation as *before*. You have a right to this information and more. If the surgeon you have chosen is patronizing or dismisses your questions, find another doctor.

If your problem is unmanageable bleeding, whether regular (cyclical) or irregular, or an unbearable sensation of discomfort or pressure, and your doctor recommends immediate surgery (without providing an acceptable and clear rationale), you might be wise to switch to someone who will seek alternatives.

> Recently, I was hospitalized for severe abdominal pain with elevated temperature, pulse, and a drop in blood pressure. It was diagnosed as PID (Pelvic Inflammatory Disease) and my gynecologist immediately recommended a hysterectomy. Uneasy about the idea of undergoing major surgery, I consulted a friend's doctor who instead suggested that, since it was the first flare-up, I try antibiotics. I was then treated with high doses of intravenous antibiotics and was released five days later. This happened four years ago this month and I've had no recurrence. I know now it pays to get a second opinion.

If you are postmenopausal and suddenly start to bleed, your doctor is even more likely to recommend hysterectomy, suspecting cancer. According to the latest statistics, this kind of bleeding is caused by cancer in only 7 percent of cases—not sufficient reason to consent to major surgery before other avenues are explored.

Some remedies for heavy bleeding are outlined in chapter 3. Aside from remedies using nonprescription drugs, a number of hormonal treatments are available: danazol (Danocrine), which is often prescribed to women with endometriosis, and GnRH or gonadotropin-releasing hormone analog (Lupron); both are prescribed to still-menstruating women in order to induce a pseudo-menopause. This treatment may be considered beneficial when endometriosis and/or fibroids cause heavy bleeding. Women who are no longer ovulating but who continue to bleed irregularly may be given progesterone (often Provera) to help flush out the uterus and tide them over until the last menstrual period. Clomiphene citrate (Clomid, the "fertility drug") is sometimes prescribed to reestablish ovulatory cycles. However, this drug stimulates growth of fibroids and should be avoided if at all possible. Because there are major side effects associated with any strong drug, it is wise to inform yourself about these before you agree to treatment. If your doctor is reluctant to discuss side effects, check the *Merck Manual* or *Physician's Desk Reference* at the library or at your pharmacist's. Another handy reference is James Long's *The Essential Guide to Prescription Drugs.*

Conditions Often Resulting in Surgery

Fibroids

The most common reason for a hysterectomy is fibroids, which are dense and harmless growths inside, outside, or between the walls of the uterus or on a stalk attached to the uterus. Fibroids are tolerable until they grow so large that they exert pressure on the rectum, bladder, or vagina—or until they cause pain during menstruation as the uterus attempts to expel them.

Fibroids are not usually dangerous. Because they thrive on estrogen, they become more troublesome as estrogen levels dip and soar just prior to menopause. Some women don't know they have fibroids until they start on ET, which causes the fibroids to grow. Once the last menstrual period has passed (assuming there is no hormone therapy), fibroids usually shrink and eventually disappear. For many women, the solution is to hold on for the last few years until menopause takes care of the situation. Should the fibroids become intolerable, a myomectomy (a procedure that removes the fibroids but not the uterus) may be possible.

Only very rarely does a fibroid become malignant

(leiomysarcoma); this is estimated to occur in one woman in 150,000. Do not be coerced into having a hysterectomy "because it might turn cancerous."

> Several years ago, my gynecologist recommended a
> hysterectomy because of a fibroid growth in my
> uterus. At the time he made no mention of alternative
> remedies, only that there seemed to be an increased risk
> of cancer if they were not removed. Terrified of even
> the thought of cancer, I underwent the surgery.
> Following the operation, I was told that he'd also
> removed both ovaries. When I asked why, he stated, "You're
> better off without them ... you have no use for them
> anyway!" Now that I know this condition could have
> been alleviated by diet, and the operation perhaps
> prevented had I had more information, it fills me with
> frustration and rage.

Fibroids may be diagnosed using a hysterogram or a sonogram. The hysterogram is frequently used if fibroids in the uterus are suspected. A dye is put into the uterus through a tube and X-rays are taken. The sonogram is a procedure using ultrasound. Either a transducer is rubbed across the belly or, in the more sophisticated procedure, a tampon-like transducer is placed inside the vagina. In order to do a sonogram, the bladder must be full, which is often uncomfortable. However, this procedure may enable you to get a more accurate diagnosis before making an important decision about taking further steps.

There is speculation that fibroids may thrive on a high-fat diet. It is known that they are much more likely to occur in women who are overweight or obese, the risk increasing with each substantial weight gain. Anecdotal information, although scientifically suspect, tells us that some women have reduced and eliminated fibroids by switching to a diet very low in fats—for example, macrobiotic or the Pritikin Diet. (Low fats may also help alleviate fibrocystic breast disease.)

Endometriosis

This condition accounts for about one-fifth of all hysterectomies. For some unknown reason, cells of the lining of the uterus (the endometrium) migrate outside the uterus and lodge inside the pelvic cavity—on the ovaries, fallopian tubes, bladder, or rectum. Slight endometriosis may go undetected because the cells are all but invisible in the early stages. However, larger clumps of cells tend to respond to the estrogen/progesterone of the normal menstrual cycle, swelling, bleeding, and causing intense pain because the blood cannot escape in the usual way. These clumps of cells eventually blacken and take on the appearance of burn sites inside the abdomen. Endometriosis is commonly found in women between the ages of thirty and forty, although it has been diagnosed in women of all ages. A woman may have to consult a number of doctors before the condition is correctly diagnosed.

Because endometriosis disappears during pregnancy, drugs that induce a false pregnancy or false menopause may provide some relief. Depending on age, a woman may be given oral contraceptives; danazol (Danocrine), a drug that mimics a weak androgen (hormone produced by the adrenal glands); or leuprolide, a GnRH or gonadotropin-releasing hormone analog (Lupron). There are potential side effects to any drug (e.g., danazol has negative effects on blood fats and GnRH analogs may affect bone strength) but it is worth investigating drug therapy before resorting to surgery. At the same time, the doctor may use laparoscopy (a fiber-optic technique) to investigate the extent of the damage.

Like a D&C, laparoscopy may be either diagnostic or operative: if the diagnosis is confirmed, cauterization or lasers may be used to burn away sites of errant cells or to remove the entire peritoneum (lining of the pelvic cavity). Laparotomy, a related but more extensive procedure, may also be indicated. Neither of these procedures will cure endometriosis but they "buy time," both for the woman who wishes to conceive and for the woman approaching natural menopause. Laparoscopy requires an overnight stay in the hospital and may be repeated with no untoward effects.

> I am thirty-six years old. Three weeks ago, I underwent surgery to remove a ten-centimeter-long cyst on my left ovary. This ovary was finally also removed as they discovered I had a severe case of endometriosis. Several cysts were also burned off the right ovary, and my doctor says I now have a 50 percent chance of recurrence, at which time my uterus, remaining ovary, and tubes will probably have to be removed—causing instant menopause.

According to the Endometriosis Association, hysterectomy is an effective remedy in only a minority of cases. Eighty-five percent of women continue to have problems after the operation, even when ET is withheld. (Many doctors suggest that ET be introduced after an interval of a few months. This means that when ovarian function is affected—as happens in one-third to one-half of cases—the patient may experience effects of menopause immediately after the operation.) If all else has failed, a hysterectomy and bilateral salpingo-oophorectomy (removal of the uterus, ovaries, and fallopian tubes) may be suggested. Even after this procedure, 5 percent of endometriosis sufferers will experience a recurrence.

Adenomyosis

This condition is similar to endometriosis and also accounts for about one-fifth of all hysterectomies. In a case of adenomyosis, endometrial cells move into the muscles of the uterus, causing the uterus to enlarge and harden. Menstruation then becomes very heavy and very painful. However, adenomyosis remains undetected in about 30 percent of cases and is discovered only when surgery is performed for another reason. Adenomyosis usually occurs in women who have had more than one pregnancy and who are between the ages of forty and fifty. It is rare after menopause.

Two years ago, I began experiencing extremely heavy bleeding during my periods. They had always been fairly light and painless but gradually I became so incapacitated by the pain, I couldn't go to work for two days each month. I was also using about three or four more tampons every day. I consulted my doctor, who suggested a D&C. He suspected I had a condition called adenomyosis so I had a hysterectomy a month later. It turned out he was right. Although my recovery has been slow and difficult, I am now better able to function and no longer have to dread that "time of the month."

Prolapse

Most of us think of *uterus* when we hear the word *prolapse*, although this is only one form of prolapse, which simply means the downward displacement of an organ or part. Prolapse may affect the uterus, the bladder, the urethra, or the rectum.

According to one well-known English doctor, about one woman in five attending her clinic has some form of uterine prolapse. This means that the uterus begins to descend into the vagina (*not* the same as a "tipped" uterus, which does not need correction). In extreme cases of prolapse, the uterus may protrude from the mouth of the vagina. Weakened pelvic muscles, as a result of childbirth or obesity, are often responsible.

The discomfort of an extreme uterine prolapse may be relieved by the insertion of a pessary, a device that lifts the uterus out of the vagina. While the pessary is in place, a

DIFFERENT TYPES OF PROLAPSE

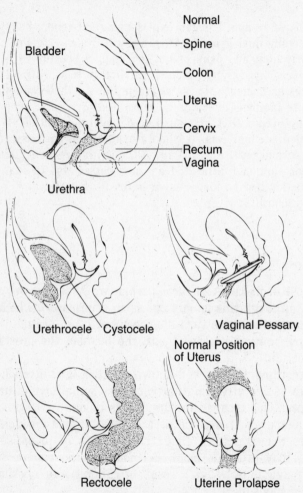

strict and regular routine of Kegel exercises should be adopted (see page 46) and, if necessary, a weight-loss program as well. Some women have found that yoga exercises are helpful, especially the shoulder stand. If this doesn't work, a minor operation called a suspension may be performed, provided the muscles are in shape. If the uterus is normal (this can be checked using an hysteroscope), surgical suspension is infinitely preferable to hysterectomy.

If hysterectomy is warranted, it will usually be done through the vagina, using the lithotomy position (similar to that used during a Pap smear), but leaving the ovaries and fallopian tubes intact; this eliminates the necessity of an incision. However, the operating table is often rotated into a near-vertical position so that the surgeon may more easily see what he or she is doing. Because the table is tilted only after the patient is anesthetized, many women wonder why they experience severe backache after the operation. This operation is also more likely to incur damage to the bladder, ureters, or to the nerves affecting bowel and bladder function than an abdominal hysterectomy. Such damage may cause the involuntary passing of small amounts of urine, which may be relieved by faithful repetitions of Kegel exercises or through a minor surgical procedure, a colporrhapy, which tightens the support around the urethra (the tube that carries urine out of the body) and takes pressure off the vaginal wall.

Prolapse, whether of the uterus, bladder, urethra, or rectum, may also be relieved by exercise and diet, before a final decision about surgery is required. Doctors have noticed that the incidence of prolapse is decreasing, perhaps because women are having fewer children or perhaps because their muscles are stronger since they are exercising more.

Cervical Abnormalities

The cervix, or bottom third of the uterus, is prone to a number of conditions which, if not watched closely or left untreated, may develop into something serious. Cervicitis is usually detected by means of an unusual discharge—unusual in color, in texture, or in aroma—a signal to make an appointment with a doctor. Or you may be told of some abnormality as the result of a routine Pap test.

Depending on the results of your Pap test, you may be referred for colposcopy. A colposcope is a special microscope that permits magnification of the cervix by ten to forty times. If suspicious cells are found, samples are scraped for biopsy. The examination takes fifteen to twenty minutes and is uncomfortable but not painful. If the biopsy is not conclusive, more tissue will be needed. Cells of the cervix may be removed using a "punch" (like the kind used to make a perforation in paper). There are no nerves in the cervix, so this is uncomfortable but not terribly painful, although severe uterine cramps may follow. (Don't plan to go back to work the same day!)

A more comprehensive sample of cells requires a *cone biopsy*, which entails a general anesthetic and hospital admission in order to remove a cone-shaped section of the cervix. This is done so that cells deeper inside the cervix can be examined. Sometimes the cone is enough to arrest any abnormality. Although some cancers of the cervix have been halted using this procedure, conization is relatively rare these days. There is a tendency for the cervix to close up as a result of the procedure, so the consequences of conization are more critical for women who wish to become pregnant. This may not be an issue for women approaching menopause. Results of the biopsy (punch or cone) vary according to the depth and extent of abnormal cells. If the abnormality is minor, a stiff brush may be enough to remove the offending cells and induce the cervix to regrow normally. If not, cryosurgery or laser surgery may be recommended.

Loop electrosurgical excision procedure (or LEEP) is a new procedure that eliminates the two steps of biopsy and then surgery. LEEP uses a low-voltage electrified wire loop to excise the tissue and thus preserve it for biopsy. This is helpful in confirming the type and extent of the abnormality, and can be performed in a matter of minutes in a doctor's office. The only concern is that the ease of the procedure may lead to abuse. Make sure that you have had a colposcopy first and that overgrowth of cells on the cervix (or CIN—cervical intraepithelial neoplasia) has been established.

In cryosurgery no anesthetic is needed. The cells on the surface of the cervix are frozen using a probe that directs a solution onto the surface of the cervix; the surface cells turn white and soon start to slough off. This procedure is uncomfortable but not painful. The process is preferable to more drastic forms of surgery, although it results in a watery discharge for days or weeks afterward, and the discharge can become foul smelling at times. But eventually the surface of the cervix grows new and normal cells.

Laser surgery, which has become increasingly popular during the last few years, vaporizes abnormal cervical tissue; it is preferred by many gynecologists who have invested in expensive laser equipment.

Each of these three procedures—LEEP, cryosurgery, and laser—is equally effective and it may be a choice that simply comes with the surgeon. It is worthwhile to inquire about the advantages and disadvantages of each, for your particular case, before consenting. This may involve talking to three different doctors.

Known risk factors for CIN are young age at first intercourse, multiple male sex partners, failure to have Pap tests, and smoking. (The nicotine found in vaginal secretions of cigarette smokers is in concentrations 40 times higher than in the blood.)

Some cervical conditions prompt remedial action, but hysterectomy is rarely warranted. Even when a diagnosis of early carcinoma in situ (malignant cells confined to the surface) is made, steps can be taken to head off further trouble, without resorting to hysterectomy. Choose your doctor carefully. Find someone with a conservative approach, someone who views major surgery as a last resort.

Pelvic Inflammatory Disease (PID)

PID is a general term used to cover a variety of inflammations that may affect the pelvic cavity. Use of an intrauterine device (IUD) for birth control, coupled with an increase in sexual activity (often with many partners) appear to have contributed to a higher incidence of PID. PID is often confused with sexually transmitted diseases (STD)—once known as venereal disease (VD)—but the causes of PID are more mysterious. It can happen to anyone. The symptoms may be pelvic pain with or without unusual bleeding but, unlike other conditions, there is often high fever during the acute phase. Most cases of PID respond to diligent treatment with antibiotics, but one episode of PID should be a signal for a woman to find and hold on to a good gynecologist. PID can lead to a higher possibility of infertility or fertility problems, usually due to scarring of the fallopian tubes. Drastic surgery may be required if PID continues.

Endometrial Abnormalities

Some women are frightened into having a hysterectomy as a result of a routine Pap test, which indicates unusual cells within the uterus. When this happens, the cells may be identified as:

- hyperplasia or hyperplastic
- cystic hyperplasia
- atypical adenomatous hyperplasia; or
- carcinoma in situ

Hyperplasia means an abnormal number of cells; this condition may occur naturally or as a result of prolonged and/or heavy use of estrogen without added progesterone. Each of these conditions is a step toward uterine cancer but none is serious enough to warrant an immediate hysterectomy. Even carcinoma in situ, frightening as it may sound, means cancerous cells that are restricted to one location; thus it may be possible to remove the cells without removing the uterus. Endometrial cancer has a high cure rate because it is extremely slow-growing. Any condition described to you as "precancerous" (or in similar words) is unnecessarily alarming. After all, there's not one cell in the entire body that isn't "precancerous."

A number of steps can be taken to change the characteristics of the endometrial cells—a course of progesterone, and one or more D&Cs. Don't assume that you are simply postponing the inevitable and agree to an unnecessary operation. Always look at the alternatives to major surgery.

> After two years without a menstrual period, I developed
> some vaginal bleeding. I had been on estrogen for
> about six years, so my gynecologist immediately
> stopped the hormones and told me to come back if there
> was any more "breakthrough bleeding" (as he called it)
> and he would do a D&C. I tried to ignore the slight
> bleeding for several months and then finally booked
> for a D&C. The results showed endometrial hyperplasia
> with atypical cells. According to the doctor, I now had
> several choices. One was to wait for more bleeding
> then another D&C and, if cells had worsened, to have
> a hysterectomy. The second choice was to have a
> hysterectomy immediately. He recommended the second
> option.
> After consulting several other doctors (including
> a young, recently graduated female gynecologist) who
> all recommended the second option, I decided to go ahead
> with the surgery. I feel a hundred percent better than

before surgery and would like to start losing weight, exercising, and being generally more careful about my health. I would also like to stop taking estrogen, which I began again after surgery, but for now it is very necessary.

I went for a six-week checkup last week and everything has healed perfectly. When I asked if I should come back for a further check, the doctor said, "There's no need to come and see me; you have nothing for me to examine."

Surgical Procedures

Dilatation and Curettage (D&C)

This minor operation is often ordered to control extensive bleeding *(menorrhagia)* when drug therapy has been unsuccessful. Dilatation opens up the uterus for inspection. The curette is a long, spoon-handled instrument that is used to scrape out the tissues lining the uterus.

A D&C may be warranted to better diagnose a problem as, for instance, following an abnormal Pap test or when adenomyosis (endometrial cells enlarging the uterus) is suspected. Sometimes a minor procedure such as this, or even a Pap test or punch biopsy may prod the uterus into regulating itself. Aside from its diagnostic value, a D&C can also relieve uterine polyps (harmless, pod-shaped growths) or submucous fibroids. If the polyps or fibroids recur, a second or third D&C may eliminate the need for major surgery.

Because the D&C is a minor procedure, it is sometimes done in an Outpatient Clinic. The patient reports early in the

DILATATION AND CURRETTAGE (D&C)

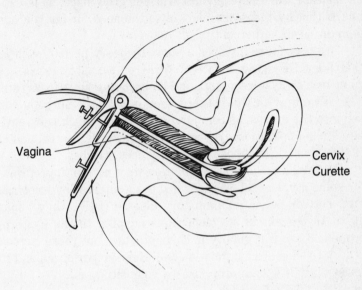

Vagina   Cervix
                                                 Curette

morning and is discharged that evening. When performed under general anesthetic, an overnight stay may be required. Scarring of the uterus may result and, for this reason, the D&C or a series of D&Cs may not be the best option for women wanting a child. For most menopausal women, however, these consequences are not so important.

Hysteroscopy and Laser Ablation

An alternative to a D&C is laser ablation of the endometrium, which may be effective when hormone treatment and/or D&Cs have been ineffective in halting severe bleeding. This procedure allows the surgeon to view the inside of the uterus using a fiber-optic device called a hysteroscope, and to destroy the deepest layer of the endometrium (lining of the uterus) either by vaporizing it with a laser or by cutting it away with a razor or a roller ball (a resectoscope). In either case, the endometrium will not grow back. It is estimated that hysteroscopy eliminates the need for further surgery in 60 to 85 percent of all cases.

This procedure involves a short recovery period (such as that for a D&C), no negative effects on sexual response (as compared to hysterectomy), and an encouraging success rate. The advantage of the hysteroscope is that the surgeon can see into the uterus, as compared to a D&C, which is essentially a blind operation. Unlike a D&C, however, destruction of the endometrium almost always induces sterility.

Hysteroscopy and laser ablation may not be appropriate for some atypical cell changes inside the uterus (hyperplasia, etc.) nor for pelvic inflammatory disease (PID). Only about 10 to 15 percent of surgeons have adapted to the hysteroscope and use it regularly in their practice, but there is good reason to shop around for someone who is experienced and to insist on it if it is appropriate to your situation.

Myomectomy

Myomectomy (or leiomyomectomy) is a procedure that is relatively rare in this country as opposed to England and western Europe, although informed health consumers are helping to make it more available. A myomectomy is an operation that removes fibroids (benign tumors known as *myomas* or *leiomyomas)* but which leaves the uterus intact. The reason it is *not* more common in North America is that doctors have been trained to think of the uterus as an unnecessary organ (except for child-bearing), and most are not trained or experienced in the myomectomy procedure, which often involves more bleeding and requires more patience, time, and attention to detail than does a hysterectomy.

FIBROIDS IN AND AROUND THE UTERUS

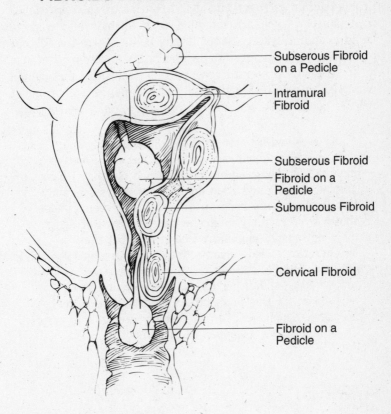

Subserous Fibroid
on a Pedicle

Intramural
Fibroid

Subserous Fibroid

Fibroid on a
Pedicle

Submucous Fibroid

Cervical Fibroid

Fibroid on a
Pedicle

Fibroids of different shapes and sizes are fairly common. About 20 to 30 percent of women harbor detectable fibroids, although only about a third will be bothered by them—experiencing abnormal bleeding, irregular menstrual periods, or feelings of pressure. Pathologists report that more than 50 percent of women have never-detected fibroids of some kind, some being so tiny as to be almost invisible during autopsy.

Surgeons who perform myomectomies remove an average of sixteen to twenty per operation, and the fibroids recur in a small minority (10 to 20 percent) of cases. However, fibroids feed on estrogen and tend to shrink as one approaches menopause. If you are troubled with fibroids and wish to avoid having a hysterectomy, it may be advisable to seek out a surgeon who will agree to perform a myomectomy. Because most surgeons prefer to reserve this procedure for women who wish to retain the possibility of pregnancy, your request will be taken more seriously if you are of child-bearing age.

I just received a letter from my sister in England; I had written to her about my upcoming surgery. Four months ago, my gynecologist informed me that I have uterine fibroids and I am due to have a hysterectomy two weeks from tomorrow. Yet my sister seems to feel that a hysterectomy might be unnecessary. She sent me a newspaper clipping which states that there is an operation called "myomectomy" that involves removing only the fibroids and not the uterus. I've since spoken to two doctors. Neither had any information about or support for this procedure. I am outraged at their attitudes! They seem to feel that my uterus is of very little importance. I happen to care about it.

Hysterectomy

The word means "removal of the uterus" although it is often (and mistakenly) used to refer to removal of the ovaries as well as the uterus. When doctors speak about a *hysterectomy* or a *TAH* (total abdominal hysterectomy), they mean removal of the uterus and cervix. A partial hysterectomy (rare in North America) removes the uterus and leaves a cervical stump. A radical hysterectomy or modified radical hysterectomy involves lymph nodes outside the uterus and often entails a longer recovery with potentially more complications.

DIFFERENT TYPES OF HYSTERECTOMY

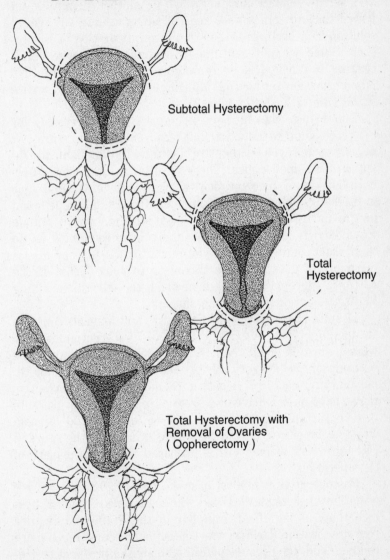

Subtotal Hysterectomy

Total
Hysterectomy

Total Hysterectomy with
Removal of Ovaries
(Oopherectomy)

Hysterectomies are performed for a number of reasons, not all valid. When three women are hysterectomized in one area of the country for every two in another, it may be inferred that hysterectomies are still being used as the "easy" solution to a problem rather than as an operation of last resort. Some women continue to assume that, once childbearing is finished, a hysterectomy is part of the routine. Misinformation or lack of information contribute to an inflated rate of hysterectomy.

Some surgeons routinely recommend a hysterectomy for heavy bleeding without attempting preliminary measures, or neglect to tell women that fibroids tend to diminish and disappear with menopause. There is often a significant difference between a male surgeon's view of your uterus and your own feelings about it. A striking example of this can be found in the hysterectomy rates in Switzerland, where female gynecologists perform half as many hysterectomies as do their male counterparts. If you feel attached to your uterus (as many of us do!), make this clear to your doctor. If the doctor is appropriate for your needs, he or she will be willing to discuss options other than surgery.

Despite the fact that medical texts and journals continue to document the adverse effects of hysterectomies, few women are told about the possibility of earlier menopause as a result of the surgery. Even when ovaries are being removed, surgeons are reluctant to mention the effects this might have on sex drive or on sexual response. Most patients believe that taking hormones will be an easy and fail-safe way to compensate for any losses resulting from the surgery. Far too many women are ill-prepared for the aftermath of the operation.

Postoperative complications affect from 10 to 25 percent of patients, particularly those who experience a radical hysterectomy. A significant number of those affected require rehospitalization. Urinary tract infections become much more common and, for premenopausal women, the prospect of premature menopause becomes a distinct possibility, a fact that

very few women are aware of. Because the ovaries are
moved inside the pelvic cavity, disrupting the blood flow
carrying essential hormones, ovarian function is often affected. High levels of estrogen circulating in the bloodstream
during the menstruating years help to protect against heart
disease and osteoporosis. When ovaries falter as a result of
hysterectomy, the risks of heart disease and osteoporosis increase.

Depression follows hysterectomy in from 30 to 50 percent
of cases—some studies say 70 percent. Usually this is a minor and short-term depression (such as after childbirth), but
it is now recognized that there is a biochemical source for
this depression. It is not due to the trauma of anesthesia or
surgery, because the effects are quite different from the experiences of women who have had appendectomies or chole-
cystectomies (gallbladder surgery).

Hysterectomy may permanently diminish the experience
of orgasm, not only because it removes the source of
prostacyclin, which is a potent vasodilator produced in the
uterus, but because it amputates the complementary throbbing of the uterus, which often accompanies orgasm. Scar tissue at the end of the vagina may inhibit the ballooning
characteristic of the vaginal barrel during orgasm; the
woman may have to use a dilator to stretch the vagina and
to plan, with her partner, sexual activity that will gradually
make intercourse more pleasurable. (If the ovaries are removed at the same time as the hysterectomy, both sexual
desire and the capacity for response may disappear.)

Estrogen can never re-create the hormonal milieu, although it works better for some women than others. Wom-
en are told that drugs will "replace" lost estrogen but not
about the high levels of gonadotropins—FSH and LH—
which appear after surgery and which may have unpredictable consequences. It is impossible to predict how effective
supplementary hormones will be for a particular patient. Nor
are women told about increased risks of osteoporosis and
heart disease that result. Most women find that it takes a full

year to feel totally well, but some spend years trying different forms of replacement therapy in an unsuccessful effort to
recapture the sensation of being well. Women are not likely
to hear much about these things from their surgeon.

If you decide to proceed with a hysterectomy, minimize
the surprises by learning as much as you can about the
operation. Recovery is often longer and more difficult if
the operation is scheduled during the two weeks prior to
menstruation, so plan accordingly. If your doctor is not particularly forthcoming, this may be the time to think about
switching. Too many women are persuaded to stick with "experienced technicians" who are incapable of communicating
effectively with their patients. Is that what you really want?
Inquire about the tests required in advance, the types of anesthetic used, the location of the incision, the pre-surgery
routine (enema? shave?), and the post-surgery possibilities
(catheter? IV [intravenous]? drains? lung expansion exercises?). Examine the release forms you will be asked to sign,
and discuss contingencies with your doctors. When might
you be expected to get up? to walk? to go home?

There are a great many women who find the quality of
life much improved after a hysterectomy and who are very
glad the decision was made. Research has shown that the
outcome of a hysterectomy is favorable when the patient has
had a few months to consider the possibilities and when she
has a very clear idea of the reasons for, and techniques used,
in the chosen procedure; the post-surgery routine; and the
detailed steps toward full recuperation. No self-respecting
surgeon objects to a second opinion, or even a third, and each
consultant is likely to contribute to a more accurate picture.

A woman who experiences extreme discomfort or continual pain will not be dissuaded by this list of "things to think
about," and rightly so. For every positive experience, however, there are many women confused and miserable after
their operations. The rate of hysterectomy is much higher
among poorly educated women with blue-collar or low-status
jobs, because these women have neither the opportunity nor

the encouragement to consider other possibilities. This is why those interested in women's health urge caution and deliberation.

Oophorectomy (or Ovariectomy)

These are the correct terms for removal of an ovary. When both ovaries are removed, the procedure is called a bilateral oophorectomy. When the fallopian tubes are also removed (as is often the case), it's called a bilateral salpingectomy—which doctors often refer to as a BSO (bilateral salpingo-oophorectomy). Women who have had this operation are known by physicians as "castrates."

Removal of all ovarian tissue causes an immediate menopause, no matter what the age of the woman. Removal of most ovarian tissue is often followed by menopause due either to the trauma (shock) of the surgery or because of a disturbance in the blood supply around the ovaries, which carries the hormones produced by ovarian tissue. This interruption to the cycle often brings on premature menopause. Theoretically one small part of the ovary can produce hormones sufficient to keep the cycle regular until natural menopause. In practice, however, the outcome is unpredictable.

Many gynecology textbooks still advocate the removal of healthy ovaries from any woman over forty. The shocking news is that this recommendation is based on a false statistic that has been published in textbook after textbook.* It's not surprising that surgeons who graduated ten, twenty, or

*In 1955, a medical text was published in which it was stated that, among women who had developed ovarian cancer, 4 to 4.5 percent had previously had a hysterectomy. In later years and later textbooks, this statistic was transposed to read that hysterectomized women stood a 4 to 4.5 percent chance of *developing* ovarian cancer. This error led to the mistaken belief that hysterectomy increased the risks of ovarian cancer and has no doubt been the rationale for the removal of countless ovaries. In fact, the risk of ovarian cancer is not affected by the presence or absence of the uterus. (Cutler, 1988:105).

thirty years ago may still adhere to this recommendation; others routinely remove ovaries when performing a hysterectomy on a woman over forty-five. This is done to avoid the possibility of ovarian cancer, a particularly lethal form of cancer that is difficult to detect and which, unlike uterine or endometrial cancer, takes hold very quickly. It is now recognized, however, that removal of the ovaries prior to natural menopause significantly increases the risks of both heart disease and osteoporosis. And the risks of heart disease and osteoporosis are incurred for *every* woman who loses ovarian tissue in order to protect the *rare* woman who will develop ovarian cancer. It is ironic that the practice of removing the ovaries in any woman over forty has led to inflated rates of heart disease and osteoporosis among older women, who are then prescribed estrogen, a medical treatment, to alleviate a condition induced by the medical procedure.

The risk of ovarian cancer in the population at large is roughly 1/100 (with the exception of families with a strong history of this disease). This risk holds for women who have had hysterectomies. There is even a suggestion that the risk may be reduced because ovaries that are found to be healthy during surgery are likely to remain healthy. Removing one healthy ovary, or all but part of one ovary, are highly questionable practices because, as long as any ovarian tissue is present, the potential for ovarian cancer remains the same.

There is considerable evidence that aging ovaries still produce testosterone (vital in maintaining sex drive and a feeling of well-being) and a substance that is converted to estrone which, in turn, helps to maintain bone strength. Choose a surgeon who is cognizant of a woman's enduring need for her ovaries. If the presence of an ovarian cyst requires investigative surgery, the patient and her surgeon should have a clear understanding that oophorectomy should not take place unless malignancy is found. This requires complete trust in your surgeon.

Prostate cancer in men is almost as common and about as lethal as cancer of the ovaries in women. However, prostectomies (the equivalent procedure for the male, which often results in impotence) are not routinely performed in order to protect them from prostate cancer. Women's health activists are protesting the practice of removing healthy ovaries.

Both hysterectomy (and oophorectomy, where warranted) may now be performed using laparoscopic surgery. This is a very new procedure which can be performed abdominally or vaginally, using small incisions in the abdomen—one through which the surgeon views the operating area, and one or more for instruments. The material to be removed (fibroids, uterus, fallopian tubes, ovaries) must be cut into pieces small enough to be removed through the incisions or through the vagina.

Very few surgeons are experienced with these techniques and not every woman will be a suitable candidate. Where appropriate, however, laparoscopic hysterectomies promise a shorter recovery period and the possibility of fewer postoperative complications.

As these new procedures become better known, women will be able to make more educated decisions and may in fact choose surgery rather than alternative, nonsurgical solutions for their gynecological problems. We hope that the growing availability of laparoscopic hysterectomy will not add to the current inflated incidence of hysterectomies and oophorectomies.

Cholecystectomy (Removal of the Gallbladder)

Gallstones are hardened bits of cholesterol, calcium, and/or bile pigments, often detected only during other surgery (often hysterectomy) or when ultrasound or CAT scans are used for some other purpose. A CAT scan may, for instance, have been ordered for suspected osteoporosis. Cholecystectomy is an operation performed three times more often on women than on men.

The gallbladder is a storage facility for bile, the enzyme that is manufactured in the liver and directed toward the small intestine to help in the breakdown of ingested fats. A gallstone may tumble into the biliary duct that transports this bile, lodge there (causing great pain), or cause an infection.

If you are overweight, over forty, and have had several children, you're in a high-risk category. Certain ethnic groups are more prone to gallstone problems (e.g., Spaniards, Swedes, Native Americans), although no one has figured out if this is due to heredity or diet. Additional risk factors are diabetes, cirrhosis of the liver (from high alcohol consumption), and use of certain types of diuretics (thiazide derivatives). Women vulnerable to gallbladder attacks are advised to stick to a low-fat diet to minimize the possibility of such an occurrence.

Pathologists tell us that one woman in five has gallstones when she dies, although they may never have given her problems. These stones may be "silent" or asymptomatic (without symptoms); doctors treat these differently from quiescent gallstones, which *do* cause symptoms that are likely to recur.

Because the risk of gallstones increases with use of oral contraceptives (particularly among very young women), oral estrogen is usually not recommended for women susceptible to gallstones. Obese women fall into this category because they already produce higher than normal amounts of estrone, a form of estrogen.

I am writing to you because I want to share my experience with other women. Last month, I was told I had gallstones and surgery was advised. After having asked around a little, I discovered that the estrogen I've been taking to deal with menopause symptoms may very well have stimulated growth of the stones. I have stopped the estrogen and have gone on a low-fat diet. So far, all is well.

THE OCCURRENCE OF GALLSTONES

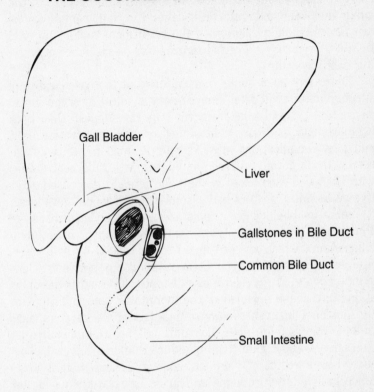

Gall Bladder

Liver

Gallstones in Bile Duct

Common Bile Duct

Small Intestine

There are a number of nonsurgical interventions for gallstones; these include pills that dissolve stones, drips that introduce a solvent directly into the gallbladder, or shock waves intended to pulverize the stones (lithotripsy), and a laparoscopic procedure. The pills have worked well on cholesterol stones, but less well on other kinds of stones (and it is impossible to analyze the stones until they are *removed).* The drip must reach the precise site of the stones (a highly specialized maneuver) because it is toxic and could damage other organs. The shock waves, which are used more successfully on kidney stones, may harm nearby lung tissue and must be done under general anesthetic. And, although laparoscopy has become popular (and easy to sell) because of the small incisions and quicker recovery period, complications are far more likely than with the traditional "open" surgical field. It pays to get precise figures on the risks accompanying each procedure.

There has been some speculation that increased rates of surgery may result from unnecessary medical intervention in asymptomatic gallstones. Recent reports suggest that both asymptomatic and quiescent stones require observation only, and that complications arise in only a small minority of patients. In one study, where candidates with quiescent stones were followed very closely, the pain actually decreased after five years. Most doctors had assumed that it would get worse.

Some gallbladder operations are recommended because of continuing flatulence (gas) and dyspepsia (heartburn/indigestion), which are presumed to be caused by gallstones. Studies have shown very little relationship between these symptoms and the presence of gallstones. Even after the operations have been performed, the symptoms tend to reappear.

The best insurance against gallbladder surgery appears to be a low-fat, high-fiber diet and vigilance to guard against excessive weight gain. (Gallbladder problems have also occurred as a result of very sudden and severe weight loss.) Since gallbladder problems appear to be related to a higher risk of heart attack, the low-fat diet advocated in Chapter 8 may help to reduce the risk of a number of diseases of midlife, including fibroids, gallstones, and breast cancer.

The prospect of surgery is rarely pleasant, and few people are wheeled in, smiling, to the operating room. It helps to have the support and counsel of someone we trust when making decisions about elective surgery. It helps, too, if the support comes from someone who understands how a woman feels about her body. Women's health organizations are doing a superb job in locating and circulating information about surgical procedures. Some are also attempting to provide an advocate for the frightened woman contemplating surgery; this advocate is a woman who will sit in on discussions with the doctor, ask pertinent questions, bolster the morale, and safeguard the rights of the woman faced with a decision. This is a role that each of us can play for one another.

REFERENCES AND RESOURCES

Aitken, J. M. et al. "Osteoporosis after oophorectomy for non-malignant disease in premenopausal women," *Brit. Med. J.*, May 12, 1973.

American Assoc. of Gynecologic Laparoscopists, 13021 E. Florence Ave., Santa Fe Springs, CA 90670-4505 (800-554-AAGL).

American Board of Medical Specialties, 1 Rotary Center, Suite 805, Evanston, IL 60201 (708-491-9091).

American Board of Obstetricians & Gynecologists, 936 North 34th St., Suite 200, Seattle, WA 98103 (206-547-4884).

American College of Obstetricians & Gynecologists, Resource Center, 409 12th Street S.W., Washington DC 20024-2188 (202-638-5577).

Amerikia, H. and T. N. Evans. "Ten-year review of hysterectomies: Trends, indications and risks," *Amer. J. Obs. Gyn.*, 134:431–437, 1979.

Cohen, S. and R. Soloway. "The epidemiology of gallstone disease," *Gallstones*. NY: Churchill Livingstone, 1985.

Curtis, L. R., G. B. Curtis, and M. K. Beard. *My Body—My Decision: What You Should Know About the Most Common Female Surgeries*. Tucson, AZ: The Body Press, 1986.

Cutler, W. B. *Hysterectomy: Before & After*. NY: Harper & Row, 1988.

Endometriosis Association, P.O. Box 92187, Milwaukee, WI 53202 (800-992-ENDO).

"Gallstones: Are there alternatives to surgery?" *Harvard Medical School Health Letter*, *12*(10), August 1987.

Freedman, E. "Hysterectomy & sexual dysfunction," *Can. J. of Ob/Gyn. & Women's Health Care*, 4:314, 1992.

Gross, A. and D. Ito. *Women Talk about Gynecological Surgery*. NY: Clarkson Potter, 1991.

Henriques, N. and A. Dickson. *Women on Hysterectomy (or How Long Before I Can Hang-Glide?)*. NY: Thorsons, 1986.

HERS (Hysterectomy Educational Resources & Services), 422 Bryn Mawr, Bala Cynwyd, PA 19004. (215-667-7757)

Hufnagel, V. (with S. K. Golant). *No More Hysterectomies*. NY: Plume, 1988.

"Hysterectomy as Social Process," *Women & Health*, *10*(1), Spring 1985.

Keyser, H. H. *Women Under The Knife: A Gynecologist's Report on Hazardous Medicine*. NY: Warner Books, 1984.

Kikku, P., Gronroos, M. et al. "Supravaginal amputation vs. hysterectomy: Effects on libido & orgasm," *Acta Obstet. Gynecol. Scand.*, 62:147, 1983.

McPherson, K. et al. "Regional variations in the use of common surgical procedures: within and between England and Wales, Canada and the United States of America," *Soc. Sci. Med.*, *15A*:273–288, 1981.

Morgan, S. *Coping with a Hysterectomy: Your Own Choice, Your Own Solutions* NY: Signet, 1985.

Napoli, M. A., ed. "An alternative to hysterectomy?" *HealthFacts* 11(84) May 1986.

Napoli, M. A., ed. "Laser surgery outclassed by a newer technology," *HealthFacts*, XVII (159); 1–5:August 1992.

National Second Surgical Program (HCFA), U.S. Department of Health & Human Services, 200 Independence Ave., SW, Washington, DC 20201 (800-638-6833 or 492-6603 MD).

Older, J. *Endometriosis: A Woman's Guide to a Common But Often Undetected Disease that Can Cause Infertility and Other Major Medical Problems*. NY: Scribner's, 1984.

Payer, L. *How to Avoid a Hysterectomy: An Indispensable Guide to Exploring Your Options Before You Consent to a Hysterectomy*. NY: Pantheon, 1987.

Randall, T. "Loop electrosurgical excision procedures gaining acceptance for Cervical Intraepithelial Neoplasia," *J. Am. Med. Assoc.* *266*(4):460–462, July 24/31, 1991.

Reidel, H. H. et al. "Ovarian failure after hysterectomy," *J. Reprod. Med.*, *31*:597–600, July 1986.

Richards, D. H. "A post-hysterectomy syndrome," *Lancet*, October 26, 1974.

Roopnarinsingh, S. and T. Gopeesingh. "Hysterectomy and Its Psychological Aftermath," *West Indian Med. J.*, 31:131, 1982.

Shainwald, S. "A legal response to hysterectomy abuse," *The National Women's Health Network News*, May/June 1985.

Simon, J. A. and G. S. diZerega. "Physiologic estradiol replacement following oophorectomy: failure to maintain precastration gonadotropin levels," *Obs. & Gyn.*, *59*(4), April 1982.

Stokes, N. M. *The Castrated Woman*. N.Y.: Franklin Watts, 1986.

Tangedahl, T.N. "Therapeutic options for gallstones," *Postgrad. Med.*, *81*(1), January 1987.

Weinstein, K. *Living with Endometriosis: How to Cope with the Physical and Emotional Challenges*. Reading, MA: Addison-Wesley, 1987.

Weiss, N. S. and B. L. Harlow. "Why does hysterectomy without bilateral oophorectomy influence the subsequent incidence of ovarian cancer?" *Amer. J. Epidem.*, *124*(5), November 1986.

8

Preparing for Menopause: Nutrition and Exercise

There are a number of ways to experience an uneventful menopause. One way is to be born into a society where menopausal ailments are virtually unknown—in a country such as Japan, for instance, where a term for *hot flashes* is nonexistent. We don't know whether this is due to culture, to race, or to diet. Another way to avoid menopausal distress would be to adhere to a well-balanced vegetarian diet, to avoid alcohol, caffeine, and cigarettes, and to be habituated to regular physical exertion. There is speculation that multiple pregnancies and long periods of breast-feeding protect against severe menopausal ailments. Perhaps the evolution of the female body is not speedy enough to adjust to the recurring menstrual cycles typical of a society that has recently learned how to use efficient contraception.

We cannot change our personal history. If we want to minimize menopausal distress, we should pay attention to nutrition and fitness before it arrives. We may also want to reconsider our attitudes toward menopause (and toward aging). The sting of menopause may not derive so much from physiological effects as from the negative connotations that we permit. Now is the time to rid menopause of its mystique, to view it as just one more rung on the ladder of life. The view from the top of the ladder is great, but you have to be fit enough to get there.

Your premenopausal years may be punctuated by a few bizarre and annoying changes that may send you to the doctor. One that bothered me, for instance, was a change in bowel movements—a change so startling that I made an appointment with the doctor and readily agreed to a barium enema. At age 45, menopause never entered my mind. Since there had been no radical changes in what I regularly ate, it never occurred to me to experiment a little to see if my body had changed its way of processing certain foods. I knew nothing about menopause and I suspect my doctor knew very little about nutrition.

> Prior to the onset of menopause, I found I was having
> problems with my digestion. I enjoyed red meat (loved
> roast beef!), lots of carbohydrates, and spicy foods.
> All of a sudden, I realized that my all-time favorites were
> giving me heartburn, indigestion, diarrhea, etc. It wasn't
> until my periods stopped that I made the connection.
> I've gradually altered my diet to include more
> vegetables, fruits, and chicken, and now have very few
> digestion problems.
>   Menopause reminds me of another, similar change
> in my life—puberty! At thirteen or fourteen, I began
> to acquire a taste for foods which I had previously disliked.
> Now, at fifty-one, my tastes are changing again. And
> there's as much to look forward to with *this* change
> of life as there was with the last one!

The basics of good nutrition are usually self-taught. Unless we have advanced training or have had a lifelong interest in diet, we probably don't know very much. We can't look to physicians for information, because medical training tends to concentrate on pathological dietary deficiencies such as scurvy or rickets. Only twenty-two medical schools in this country require a course in nutrition and, of those schools offering an elective in nutrition, only 5 percent of medical students register. Thus it is not surprising that so few doctors consider diet when seeking solutions to a medical problem. Dietitians, on the other hand, view proper nutrition as the sane approach to the prevention of a host of modern-day malaises, and recent cross-cultural data (gleaned by epidemiologists) have added weight to this perspective. Diet appears to be the major factor in the low incidence of breast cancer among Japanese women and the virtual absence of cardiovascular disease among the Inuit of northern Canada.

Not only must we be reeducated in terms of nutrition, but we must also take a whole new look at the benefits of exercise. For too long, physical activity has been considered to be a distasteful way of losing inches—and perhaps pounds. During the past twenty years, however, we have witnessed a revolution—exercise as the route to fitness rather than solely as a way of slimming. Women who have incorporated exercise into their lives discover that they can't do without it. More and more, exercise is proving to be the panacea we have been looking for—a way to reduce the intensity of hot flashes, to ward off the effects of depression, to find time to be by oneself, to keep one's weight at a sensible level, to help insure restorative sleep, to prevent the ravages of osteoporosis, and to minimize the risks of cardiovascular disease. The relationship between diet/exercise and maintenance of good health becomes more and more evident. If menopause is on *your* horizon and you want to manage it well, there is a great deal you can do to prepare for it.

Nutrition in Midlife

I have weighed between 130 and 135 pounds since I was about twenty-five years old. I am now forty-nine. Two

years ago, my weight soared—within a period of five
months—to 170. Needless to say, I was devastated, and
set out to find an appropriate diet. Until six months ago,
absolutely nothing helped. I tried almost every diet
I could get my hands on. I spoke to two doctors, both
of whom said, "Menopause," but neither offered any help.
They seemed to feel it was biologically inevitable and
that I'd simply have to get used to weighing thirty-
five pounds more. Finally, I decided to see a
nutritionist. This woman has taken the time to explain
to me the various changes that are happening and she
created a personalized diet for me, including my likes
and dislikes, and making sure that I get the proper
amounts of vitamins and other key nutrients. After four
months on this diet, I've lost 15 pounds and am feeling
much better.

Caloric needs decline by 2 percent per decade after the
age of twenty. This means the average woman in her forties
(height 5'4", weight 120) needs about 1900 calories per day;
this will dwindle to 1800 as she approaches age fifty. Because
we need fewer and fewer calories as we age, now is the time
to learn about "nutrient-dense" foods, and to evaluate cus-
tomary intake of foods rich in vitamins A, B, and C, as well
as riboflavin and folic acid. This is particularly important if
alcohol is part of our routine, because alcohol inhibits the
positive benefits of some vitamins and supplies "empty calories."

Vitamins A, B, and C have been found to be inadequate in
the diets of many menopausal women, and these diets have
probably been inadequate for some years. Vitamin B_2 (riboflavin) and folic acid (from green, leafy vegetables) are related to optimum cognitive function. Because forgetfulness is
a common aggravation during menopause, you can minimize
the possibility by improving your diet. Your need for iron is
lessened as the reproductive years draw to a close (so you
can forget about *ever* learning to like liver!), but you would

be wise to wean yourself away from sugar in your decaffeinated coffee, and to reduce your sodium intake.

Caffeine may not keep you awake now, but many of us
have belatedly discovered that it began to play a part in
sleeplessness or early-morning awakening as we got older.
Caffeine also blocks the absorption of calcium needed for
strong bones, of some B vitamins, of iron, and of vitamin A.
Caffeine may be responsible for a tendency to breast cysts
and, as you get closer to the last menstrual period, often acts
as a trigger for hot flashes. For diehard caffeine-addicts (I
was one), the potency of the product is directly related to the
pain of withdrawal. If you drink a lot of coffee, tea, and/or
cola drinks, giving them up may bring on a severe and prolonged headache, but this usually passes within a few days.

The good news is that there are many palatable decaffeinated beverages—including espresso, brewed or filtered coffees, and delicious herbal teas. Those of us who have made
the switch (after years of procrastinating) try to avoid restaurants that serve packets of instant coffee with a cup of
hot water, and always make a point of asking for brewed decaffeinated. (Maybe eventually they'll get the message!) The
rumors about decaffeinated coffees being carcinogenic
(cancer-causing) when treated with methylene chloride to remove the caffeine seem to be just that—rumors. The Swiss
water process and the use of ethyl acetate avoid this risk, so
read labels. Many restaurants also offer herbal teas, some of
which are caffeine-free. Ask to see the package.

Drinking black coffee (decaffeinated, that is) or clear tea
(herbal, of course) requires three weeks of disciplined effort.
After the taste buds are retrained, coffee or tea with sugar
is like drinking syrup—fine with pancakes but too sweet as
a beverage. Refined sugar contributes to the potential for
high blood pressure, tends to block the benefits of some B vitamins (thiamine, riboflavin, choline, and niacin), and contributes to the incidence of nonspecific vaginitis. Because we
become more and more prone to vaginal infection as we approach and pass the last menstrual period, the absence of re-

fined sugar is a preventive against such infections, as well as against dental cavities and weight gain.

The use and overuse of salt is related to incipient high blood pressure, a condition that affects more women than men. Many women also find that it contributes to "bloat"—the unexpected and often grotesque swelling of the abdomen, which can cause extreme discomfort. Salt is an acquired taste, and most prepared foods (packaged soups and fast foods) are heavily salted to suit the taste of Americans. Learning to do without extra salt is easier than it sounds. Lemon juice or combinations of herbs and spices are welcome substitutes, and there are many salt substitutes on the market.

The big breakthrough in nutritional research involves fat. Changes in our diet during the last half century have included enormous increases in the proportions of fats consumed as part of the so-called normal diet. It is now widely believed that a sharp reduction in the amounts and types of fat in our diet can significantly affect our predisposition to many forms of cancer, as well as to cardiovascular disease—coronary heart disease, angina, stroke, congestive heart failure, and hardening of the arteries.

Although many of us switched from butter to margarine long ago (at least at home) and reduced the consumption of eggs and fried foods in an effort to reduce dietary cholesterol, we are now told that this was either not enough or totally unnecessary (depending on whom you listen to). Many nutritionists would like us to cut down on meat (containing about 1 mg of cholesterol per gram) and eggs (containing about 250 mg each) to hold dietary cholesterol at from 250 to 300 mg per day. This can be compared to an intake of 400 mg of cholesterol per day in the average North American diet.

The information about cholesterol has been confusing because of the continuing debate about two key issues. One has to do with how cholesterol is processed by the body—how much of the cholesterol in the bloodstream is produced inside the body and how much is a result of cholesterol in the foods we eat. The other issue is the discovery that one-third to one-fifth of the population has a genetic tendency to high blood cholesterol. Until this condition was recognized, it was thought that *all* high cholesterol levels resulted from diet.

I am one of those women who has a genetic tendency to high blood cholesterol. In my case, it is due to a deficiency in cholesterol receptors—a 50 percent deficiency! I've had a dangerously high level of cholesterol for at least 20 years (260 mg/dl of blood) and, over these years, no amount of diet control has been able to lower the level significantly. Over the last six months, however, a new combination of drugs has lowered it dramatically. I now feel I can look forward to a healthy level of cholesterol and even a gracious old age!

Nowadays, if a family tendency to high cholesterol levels is discovered (usually during routine medical checkups), potential problems can be offset to some degree by scrupulous attention to diet and carefully supervised medication.

A few years ago, serum cholesterol levels—expressed, as above, in milligrams per deciliter of blood—of 240 mg/dl were considered critical. A woman with TC (total cholesterol) of 265 mg/dl was considered to be at twice the risk of cardiovascular disease as compared to someone with a TC of 205 mg/dl. Now the emphasis has moved to a concern about the ratio of HDLs to TC, the ratio of LDLs to HDLs, and the level of triglycerides.

Cholesterol circulates through the system, carried by fat molecules. Some of these fats, known as HDLs (high density lipoproteins), act to flush cholesterol and LDLs (low density lipoproteins) out of the blood vessels. LDLs carry cholesterol into target organs, depositing it on artery walls. If LDL levels are too high, circulation clogs and clots are formed—precursors to hypertension, heart disease, and stroke. In men, the risks are associated with *both* low HDLs and high LDLs. In women, the crucial factor seems to be HDL levels, so more and more emphasis is being placed on keeping HDLs high in women at risk.

The level of HDLs (ideally, over forty) and ratio of HDLs to total cholesterol (expressed as TC/HDL) is a routine index of heart health. A ratio of 3 is excellent, meaning that HDLs constitute one-third of blood cholesterol. The ratio for the average woman is 4.5. To evaluate your own heart health, arrange for a standard blood test measuring cholesterol, lipid, and triglyceride levels. You should fast for twelve hours and avoid strenuous exercise for twenty-four hours before such a test. You need to know total blood cholesterol (TC), levels of HDLs and LDLs, *and* triglyceride levels (see page 139). Total cholesterol divided by HDL, ideally, should be less than 4.0. LDLs divided by HDLs should be less than 3.0. Triglyceride levels under 200 to 250 mg/dl are normal, 250 to 500 is borderline, and 500 mg/dl is too high.*

If your test results are worrisome, there's a lot of help available which will enable you to change your eating habits. The link between low fats and low heart disease and cancer rates was first noticed in countries that habitually consume foods low in fat. It is estimated that about 40 percent of the average diet in this country consists of fat and that, to insure against a host of health risks, this should be reduced by at least 10 percent, preferably more. People who consistently adhere to a low-fat diet have been found to have reduced rates of many kinds of cancer—colorectal, prostate, breast, mouth, throat, larynx, and esophagus.

Fats in the bloodstream are hazardous not only because of the deposits inside the arteries but also because of the action of free radicals. Free radicals, which are thought to interfere with the body's defenses against cancer, are molecules that can start a chain reaction, rupturing cell

---

*Premarin at .625 mg daily over a period of three months will increase HDLs by an average of 16 percent, but will also increase triglyceride levels by 24 percent. The Estraderm patch does not raise HDLs or triglycerides.

membranes and crippling the body's ability to marshal cancer-preventing nutrients.

> I was diagnosed as having breast cancer three years ago. Since then, I've undergone surgery and radiation therapy. It appears the cancer is now in remission. Although I'm sure the radiation has had an impact on the cancer, I wanted to tell you about the role that diet has played in my situation. Immediately after my surgery, the doctor recommended I see a dietitian. I was told to keep track of which foods and how much I'd eaten for two weeks. I subsequently discovered that my diet was very high in fats and that this may have had some influence on the development of cancer.
>
> In my case, the genetic tendency was strong (my mother died of breast cancer), but the importance of nutrition in decreasing the risks was brand new to me. I'm not only eating better now but, more important, I am extremely conscious of the role of diet in the (hopefully permanent) remission of this disease.

Free radicals are constantly being produced in the body, not only in response to certain foods but as a result of pollutants in the air and other environmental factors. We cannot eliminate free radicals, but we can reduce them, and it is believed that the metabolism of fats produces the most damaging radicals. A reduction in fat intake allows the body's own defenses to mobilize and overcome any threat posed by roaming free radicals.

Obviously one cannot eliminate fats altogether, so it is helpful to know about various kinds of fat. Nutritionists recommend that saturated fats constitute no more than 10 percent of daily calories and that polyunsaturated (or monounsaturated) fats constitute no more than 10 percent. Saturated fats include butter, cheese, beef, veal, pork, coconut, and palm oils. Coconut and palm oil are often disguised as "vegetable oil" in prepared mixes and toppings. Polyunsaturated fats, including mayonnaise, margarine, and corn, sunflower, and safflower oils, are fine at room temperature but, when heated, produce the free radicals thought to damage artery walls. If you want to avoid both saturated fat and the dangers of free radicals released by hot polyunsaturates, use monounsaturated fats such as olive oil or peanut oil. Or do fat-free cooking in a non-stick pan. Holding the line at 10 percent saturated plus 10 percent poly- or monounsaturated may *appear* to permit only 20 percent fats, but experts tell us that there is likely to be another hidden 10 percent consumed daily.

The dangers of red meat (as sources of both cholesterol and fat) are still very real despite the beef industry's aggressive advertising to recapture favor. Unfortunately, the advertising doesn't respond to some basic concerns about current livestock practices. Many of us have read about the Puerto Rican children whose precocious sexual development has been traced to high levels of DES (a synthetic estrogen) fed to beef cattle. Estradiol (another form of estrogen), progesterone, and testosterone (the male hormone) are routinely fed to livestock—as are antibiotics, plastic hay, newsprint and cardboard (for roughage), and oral larvicides. Given our ignorance about the long-term consequences of these chemicals in the food chain, it is not surprising that many people choose to limit their intake of beef, pork, and veal. In other words, there is more than fat and cholesterol involved.

Vegetarians benefit from the absence of meat in their diets. Not only do they develop strong bones (vegetarians rarely suffer from osteoporosis), but the emphasis on fresh vegetables and fresh fruit provides the kind of fiber that keeps the stomach and intestinal tract healthy. High-fiber diets appear to protect against heart disease, diverticulitis, and colon cancer, and help to avoid the kinds of problems with indigestion and constipation that are so often linked to aging.

Chicken and fish become more appealing as we age—perhaps an instance of "wisdom of the body." Because chicken fat resides on the skin, it is easily removed, and the oilier fishes appear now to confer hidden benefits in terms of heart-protecting fatty acids. I spent years pushing fish around my plate every Friday at dinner, but now I order fish almost every time I eat out. I have found that fresh fish (and swift delivery from sea to market) makes an enormous difference, persuading me to forget an ancient grudge and to experiment with the wide range of fish available. And although I don't care to handle raw fish, it's one dish that cooks up evenly and quickly in a microwave.

It is difficult to make sudden changes in the diet, because such changes often involve new ways of cooking and new recipes to replace familiar dishes that we're used to preparing. For example, I find it virtually impossible to add up grams of fat or milligrams of calcium, not to mention caloric values. If your number memory is as poor as mine, it is helpful to check lists of foods and then to remember the *foods* that you should be eating.

I have been meeting more and more people who have seen a nutritional consultant either to lose weight or simply because they want to know more about the subject. Although the terms *dietitian* and *nutritionist* are used almost interchangeably, there *can* be a difference. Registered Dietitians (RDs) complete an undergraduate or graduate degree with a program in dietetics or nutrition and also complete an approved practical program or internship. Someone who calls him- or herself a *nutritionist* or *nutritional consultant* may or may not be a dietitian, may be trained in food sciences, in biochemistry, in naturopathy—or it may mean someone with a particular interest in health food publications (many of which run advertisements for mail-order degrees). If you want sound advice about what you eat and how it may affect your health, make sure you know with whom you're dealing.

Until you get interested enough to formulate your own rules, here are some basic guidelines that will help you to get healthy for menopause:

- Reduce consumption of refined sugar, salt, and alcohol.
- Eliminate caffeine.
- Watch out for the tannin in tea and red wine.
- Get in the habit of drinking water; aim for 6 to 8 glasses a day.
- Eat lots of whole-grain cereals and breads, and brown rice.
- Eat lots of fresh fruits and vegetables, preferably raw or very slightly cooked. (Store raw, cut vegetables in covered airtight containers.)
- Eat fish twice a week. Eat broiled chicken (skin removed) at least once a week.
- Explore meat substitutes (tofu, soya beans) or vegetarian dishes.
- Use small amounts of butter for frying; use peanut oil in wok cooking; use nonstick cookware for frying.
- Try low-fat dressings, dips, sauces (natural yogurt instead of sour cream, etc.)
- Drink 4 cups of skim milk or equivalent daily (containing less than one-fifth the fat content of 2 percent milk.)
- Avoid bacon, cured or processed meats, or meat spreads. (Nitrites in these foods promote free radicals.)
- If you chew gum, make sure it's sugar-free.

It would take a saint to make all of these changes at once and make them stick. However, just doing a few is a good start. Like all good habits, healthy eating takes practice, backsliding, and more practice.

Keeping Fit

Exercise is probably the most necessary and most overlooked prescription for a problem-free menopause. Exercise builds strong bones and tones up the cardiovascular and respiratory systems, reducing the risks of osteoporosis, arthri-

tis, emphysema, hypertension, heart disease and stroke.*
Exercise has also been found effective in treating depression,
constipation, and insomnia, and in guarding against the hor-
rors (!) of midlife weight gain. Exercise appears to increase
the body's capacity to perspire, and the ability to sweat appears to be related to the ability to tolerate fluctuations in
temperature. (A Swedish study found that women who exercise regularly and vigorously rarely have severe hot flashes.)
Regular exercise is associated with a 33 percent reduction in
the risk of diabetes (noninsulin-dependent diabetes mellitus).
The incidence of breast, uterine, and cervical cancer is substantially reduced among women athletes. And exercise is a
great way to avoid constipation and the hemorrhoids that
sometimes result.

Exercise has proven beneficial for older women confined
to wheelchairs; for example, regularly squeezing a tennis ball
increased the strength of their arms. Unless there are valid
medical reasons *not* to exercise, we should all be enjoying
regular physical activity. Why then do so few of us exercise?

For too many women, exercise is anything but routine. It
is something that is added to the daily (or weekly) schedule
when circumstances—time, money, relationships—permit.
This means that any sustained positive feelings derived from
exercise are rarely experienced, or experienced for only a
short time before being put aside in favor of other demands.
Women over fifty who have exercised on a regular basis
throughout their adult lives are rare. (Women over sixty are
pearls!) I don't think it is coincidental that many nonexer-
cisers have a difficult menopause.

When the Melpomene Institute, an organization devoted
to research in women's health, conducted an informal survey
of their membership to discover the reasons given for *not*

---

*In a comparative study of health status among women who had attended
the same college, the women who had *not* been actively engaged in athletics
were found to have 86 percent more breast cancer and were 153 percent more
likely to have developed uterine or cervical cancer as compared to their class-
mates who had been active in college athletics.

being physically active, more than 90 percent of the responses involved lack of time—either demanding jobs or
overwhelming family responsibilities. But some women gave
more than one reason for not undertaking regular exercise.
One woman in five was afraid that she wouldn't perform well;
one in six cited a lack of encouragement from others or the
influence of persons who felt that she shouldn't be athletic.
One in ten was influenced by others who felt that she
couldn't be athletic. Only a small minority was held back by
the perceived cost involved; far more were restrained by past
or future opinions of others, whether real or anticipated.
Close to 20 percent had *no* excuse for lack of physical activity.

I want to share my experience. When I hit menopause,
I immediately gained fifteen pounds. Weight gain was
not unusual for me, but this time it all went to my
middle instead of clinging to my hips and thighs as it
usually does. I realized that I was dealing with a different
kind of animal and that I better do something. I
checked out a few health clubs in my area but felt
like too much of an old bat to join one. I'd never been
athletic and got uncomfortable merely at the thought
of how I'd look in a leotard! Finally, I watched a class
at the local Y and found the class for me. It's a low-
impact aerobic class given in the mid-afternoon. I have
a part-time job (mornings only), so it's great. Apart from
two to three young mothers who put us all to shame,
the class is made up largely of women in their forties
or fifties who are afflicted with the same kind of midlife
bulge as me. We laugh at ourselves and cheer each other
on. Although I've only lost a few pounds, I've made
some wonderful new friends and feel better than ever.

Despite the range of benefits that accrue to heart, lungs,
blood vessels, bones, joints, brain, and self-image, regular exercise requires only three basic components—a warm-up, an
aerobic period, and a cool-down.

The warm-up is a five- to ten-minute period of stretching, which helps to prevent injury during the more active part of the exercise. If you have ever taken part in a dance, fitness, or aerobics class, you will recognize the warm-up. But this warm-up should precede *every* kind of active exercise— before stepping onto the tennis or badminton court, or pushing off on your bicycle. If you swim, you can do stretching exercises in the shallow water before you start swimming laps. This preparation will ensure that your muscles are warm and supple. Many of the exercise tips that we learned years ago—limbering movements on first awakening, the first poses of a yoga class—fulfill this function. Vital as they are, however, they are not enough.

The core of regular physical activity is the *aerobic exercise*, a term that means the kind of strenuous exertion that carries oxygen into the system and gets your pulse beating at a sustained rate over a period of at least twenty minutes. Aerobic exercise may include dancing, jogging, skipping, cross-country skiing, cycling, rowing, or brisk walking—any exercise that is uninterrupted and that pushes you to concentrated exertion. Most racket sports are not particularly aerobic, but squash and handball (which involve more continuous effort) are more aerobic than tennis or badminton. (And championship levels of any racket sports *can* be aerobic.) Swimming is aerobic only if the swimmer is going "all out" for a sustained period of time. Swimming laps may be relaxing and, to a degree, bone-strengthening, but the benefits for cardiovascular fitness are debatable. Brisk walking and cycling can be both aerobic and bone-building, but more beneficial to the legs than to the upper body. (Jogging and power or fitness walking require involvement of the arms as well.) Yoga or t'ai chi are not aerobic, although they increase flexibility and reduce stress.

It is the aerobic component of exercise that is directly beneficial to heart, lungs, and (if involving weight-bearing activity) to the bones. The aerobic component requires the most discipline, pushing oneself to breathe more efficiently (in through the nose, out through the mouth) and to perform

better and longer, time after time. Because the aerobic component *is* demanding, it is recommended that every woman
have a thorough physical examination before embarking on
any aerobic activity program.

To judge whether you have had a good workout, you need
to take your pulse. This can be done either in the standard
way, using the wrist, or by placing your fingers under the
jaw just below the ear. Count the number of beats over fifteen seconds and multiply by 4. You should be aiming for a
pulse rate of 220 minus your age times .75. (The .75 signifies
75 percent of maximum heart rate.) In other words, if you are
forty-five, you should aim for a pulse rate of 131 per minute:

$$220 - 45 = 175 \times .75 = 131$$

If you are *beginning* aerobics and are over fifty, it is recommended that you look for a pulse rate of 60 percent of maximum heart rate. Using the same formula as above, this
would be:

$$220 - 50 = 170 \times .60 = 102$$

In time, the heart rate should be raised to around 126.

If you stop moving, the heart rate starts to plummet. If
you want to monitor heart rate while exercising, slow down to
a walk (don't stop), take a quick count for six seconds, and
add a zero. Exceeding 80 percent of your maximum heart rate
is not advisable. Once you have been doing aerobic exercise
for a few weeks, you should be able to get your pulse rate up
to the desired level and hold it there for twenty minutes. A
lower pulse rate means you're not working hard enough.

After the aerobic exercise, you need a short period of
time to cool down, but be sure to wind down slowly. This is
often the most overlooked aspect of an exercise program. A
sudden stop is not good for the body, so walk around for a
few minutes and allow your muscles to cool down. Then use
a mat or folded blanket and stretch some more. Fitness instructors often add mat work to the cool-down, which may
take twenty minutes or more of an hour-long class. However,

the cool-down, like the warm-up, need last no more than five to ten minutes.

Experts suggest a minimum of three exercise sessions per week, with an optimum of five. Strenuous exercise every day of the week is not necessary and, in fact, may be harmful.

Time of day is up to you, but you should avoid eating just before exercise. If you have trouble getting to sleep, a brisk walk after dinner (not too close to bedtime) may alleviate the problem. If you work from nine to five, you may want to schedule your exercise for early morning, during the lunch hour, or immediately after work. Investigate the kinds of facilities available in the area around your work and home. In many centers, there are free-lance fitness instructors who will lead a class if you can organize a group and find a suitable place. The new low-impact exercises avoid the strain that high-impact aerobics place on the knees and ankles, and are also less noisy.

If you find group exercise abhorrent, there are alternatives, but it requires dedication to get your heart rate up and keep it there. One suggestion is to get a pedometer and a Walkman (or a friend) and start a walking program. If you use a Walkman, make your own tapes, starting off slowly (with stretching exercises at home), then warm-up walking, building up to a brisk pace that encourages you to pump your arms, and then slowing down again. If you walk with a friend, arrange to meet somewhere equidistant from your homes so that you can avoid the temptation to beg off during inclement weather.

In my city, there is a hiking organization which organizes hikes every Sunday in three categories: easy, medium, and difficult. Their fee is $5 for the day. I started by going on the easy hikes, afraid I wouldn't be able to make it. But it wasn't many months before I was going on the medium hikes. I wasn't first up the hill, but I got

there! Then I met the man I married and we began
going on our own hikes and climbs.

My husband is a member of the Alpine Club. He
introduced me to rock climbing and the use of ropes.
I enjoy it but you don't have to rock climb in order
to get exercise. A good hike up a mountain, taking small
steps at a steady pace, and not stopping until you have
gone for an hour (and then resting), is an excellent
way to get uninterrupted exercise which pushes you
to concentrated exertion. And not only that—all around
you is the beauty of nature and you are breathing in
fresh air, not car fumes. And when you get to the
top, there is the view and out comes your lunch and
flask of herbal tea. What a feeling of satisfaction!

Many women feel they can get enough activity by following TV exercise programs or videotaped workouts. The problem with these is that they are either too short to bring the
heart rate up for any sustained period of time or they get bor-
ing very quickly, or both. The same can be said for exercycles
and skipping in place. They may be adequate for highly disciplined types who will take the time to cycle, jog, or skip in
place, but most of us don't have that kind of dedication.

Women who are busy and who must cope with heavy demands at work and at home are often (and understandably)
reluctant to commit themselves to sessions of frantic aerobics, and are more attracted to the relaxation of hatha-yoga
or t'ai chi. These are marvelous adjuncts to exercise, but
they don't give your heart a workout. If you are competitive
by nature, you will find that the effort to keep up with a
good aerobics instructor is just what you need to take a
break from your problems. Because you have to concentrate
on the coordination of feet, arms, and breathing, you get a
good 40 minutes off from everyday worries.

Most of the articles and books about fitness and physical
conditioning imply and sometimes even *promise* that exercise will restore or maintain a youthful body. This claim is

misleading. You may or may not lose weight, but exercise has a value beyond any change in silhouette or dress size.

As we age, excess weight is deposited on different body parts. Through the thirties and forties, we fret about weight on the hips and thighs. As we enter the fifties, our waistlines and abdomens start to spread, and chest size (and often bra size) may increase. The rib cage is at its broadest between the ages of fifty-five and sixty-four. Most of these tendencies are inherited, so you probably know what to expect. Exercise may delay bodily changes due to aging, but there is no way that it can turn back the hands of the clock.

There is also a tendency to accumulate fat as we age. The body of a typical twenty-year-old woman consists of just over 25 percent fat; in the thirties and forties this increases to 33 percent and, by the fifties, to over 40 percent. Some increase in the proportion of body fat is bound to occur despite regular rigorous exercise. Even competitive women athletes (who can safely reduce body fat to no *less* than 12 percent of body weight) find that it takes longer and harder workouts to stay in shape. Physical activity will enhance a feeling of well-being for the average woman; it cannot obliterate the normal effects of age.

Nor is this all bad. As mentioned in chapter 3, women who are 10 to 15 pounds over "ideal weight" suffer less from severe hot flashes. (And remember that hot flashes often start a year or two before the last menstrual period.) According to the Gerontology Research Center of the National Institute on Aging, weight gain is a normal result of aging, and mortality rates are *lower* for women who are slightly overweight based on standard weight/height charts.

To use their formula for calculating height and weight, divide height (in inches) by 66, multiply the result by itself, and then multiply this result by your age plus 100. Let's assume you are 45 and 5′4″ tall: 64 (inches) divided by 66 = .969; .969 × .969 = .939; .939 × 145 (age plus 100) = 136 pounds. You can add or subtract 9 pounds to allow for light or heavy bone structure, but this will give you a significantly higher weight than the conventional Metropolitan Life Insurance tables.

An alternative way of gauging healthy weight is the Body Mass Index (or BMI), which is being used in many articles about weight. This is weight in kilograms (2.2 lb. = 1 kg) divided by height in meters (12 in. = .3048 of a meter) squared, or kg/m^2. An easier way of using the BMI is to plot your weight on the Body Mass Index chart shown on the facing page. Find your height on line A and your present weight on line B. Draw a line through these two points and extend it to line C. If the line you draw intersects line C between 20 and 25, you are in the "normal" range—which is the range designated as producing the lowest health risks. If the index reveals a number below 20 or above 27, you are at increased risk for a number of health problems. If line C is bisected at 30 or above, you are medically "obese."

Both of these newer ways of calculating weight allow for a more realistic profile and shift the emphasis away from pounds to fitness. Regular exercise may tone you and trim away inches, but may *not* trim away pounds. It will lead to cardiovascular fitness, improved muscle tone, a firmer body, and can help maintain body weight. What more do you want?

Those of us who have given up smoking recognize that added weight is the price one often pays for cleaner lungs and increased life expectancy. Ex-smokers who smoked fewer than ten cigarettes a day may gain only about 5 pounds; those who smoked a pack or more a day may have to accept a heavier weight gain. This is not such a terrible price to pay for the health gains of *not* smoking, not to mention the benefits of once again being part of a majority!

Because so many groups are available to help one stop smoking, it seems unnecessary to preach about the evils of smoking. We know that smokers are prone to high calcium loss (resulting in brittle bones), increased risks of lung cancer, emphysema, asthma, heart disease, and stroke, and earlier menopause. It is said that giving up smoking is worse than

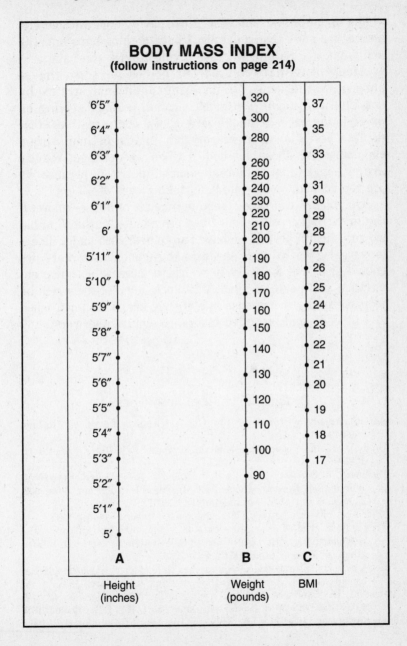

BODY MASS INDEX
(follow instructions on page 214)

| A
Height
(inches) | B
Weight
(pounds) | C
BMI |

giving up heroin—I believe it! Now, having done without cigarettes for more than a decade, I have nothing but sympathy and support for those who are trying to kick the habit.

Many of us have abused our bodies for some time—abused in the sense of imposing additional strains by smoking, consuming too much alcohol, perhaps relying on prescription drugs (tranquilizers or oral contraceptives) that deplete essential nutrients or that inhibit optimum brain chemistry. We abuse our bodies when we don't get regular exercise and when we forego sensible nutrition because we are too rushed, or too intent on taking care of others.

Our bodies can take a certain amount of abuse—more, if the first two decades of our lives provided a "cushion" of basic good health; less, if we have had to deal with major illness or surgery. As we look ahead to the menopausal years, we should also look for ways in which to increase stamina, endurance, and peace of mind. With luck, none of these will be jeopardized by menopause but, if they are, a well-nourished and fit body will be added insurance against the worst.

REFERENCES AND RESOURCES

AICR (American Institute for Cancer Risks) Nutrition Hotline: 800-843-8114.

Brody, J. E. "Exercise is the fountain of youth," *NY Times*, June 10–11, 1986.

Dickinson, A. *Safety of Vitamins and Minerals: A Summary of the Findings of Key Reviews*. Council for Responsible Nutrition, Suite 602, 2100 M Street N.W., Washington, DC 20037.

"Focus on Physical Activity," *The Melpomene Report*, October 1985.

Frisch, R. E. et al. "Lower prevalence of breast cancer and cancers of the reproductive system among former college athletes compared to non-athletes," *Brit. J. Cancer, 52*(5):885, 1985.

Lock, M. ed. "Anthropological Approaches to Menopause: Questioning Received Wisdom," *Culture, Med. & Psychiat, 10*(1), March 1986.

Luce, G. G. "Exercises for Vitality and Flexibility," in *Your Second Life: Vitality & Growth in Middle and Later Years*. NY: Delta Books, 1979.

The Melpomene Institute, *The Bodywise Woman*. NY: Prentice Hall, 1990.

Mindell, E. *The Vitamin Bible.* NY: Warner Books, 1979.

Pritikin, N. & P.M. McGrady, Jr. *The Pritikin Program for Diet and Exercise.* NY: Bantam, 1979.

Prudden, B. *Bonnie Prudden's After Fifty Fitness Guide.* NY: Ballantine, 1986.

Shephard, R. J. "Exercise and the aging process: Prescribing a programme," *Geriat. Med., 1,* October 1985.

Walsh, B. W., I. Schiff, B. Rosner et al. "Effects of postmenopausal estrogen replacement on the concentrations and metabolism of plasma lipoproteins," *New Engl. J. Med., 325:*1196–1204, 1991.

9

Relationships at Midlife

Life can get complicated for the menopausal woman. If her body is being buffeted by wayward hormones, she wants a predictable routine, not too much stress, and the sympathetic support of her friends and her family. Too often, the man in her life is more exasperated than sympathetic, and many women, resenting the lack of interest or concern, decide to keep their problems to themselves. But the man may also be dealing with his own demons—a nagging sense of "Is that all there is?," a diminishing sex drive, ambivalence about impending retirement coupled with a determination to tough it out until the best possible pension is assured.

The menopausal mother may also be dealing with inconsiderate teenagers (is there any other kind?) or with young adults who leave home, only to return weeks or months later, adding yet one more element of unpredictability to her life. Or she may find that her home is suddenly empty. There may be aging parents who need her to run errands, to do shopping, to accompany them to the doctor. And today, on top of all this, she is likely to be holding down a full-time job.

If a woman is feeling well, these various demands can

sometimes be juggled quite successfully. If she is not feeling well, the pressure can be overwhelming. It helps to know that it is happening to others. It helps to discuss the situation with friends because, by talking it over, you can often sort out which demands on your time should take priority and why. Remember, this too shall pass.

Female Friendships

It's unfortunate that many of us have to wait until our forties or fifties to cherish the commonsense advice and support we receive from our female friends. Our single friends have learned to value their married women friends, and many of the newly divorced or widowed quickly relearn the value of friends, but too many married women make room for female friendships only in the spaces not occupied by husbands and children. I'm sorry that I waited so long to find time for my friends—meeting for dinner, meeting for a weekend at a country inn, making impromptu long-distance calls just to keep in touch. Once upon a time, those of us without dates on a Friday or Saturday night would congregate for an evening of talk about life, love, and the pursuit of happiness. For many of us, that was the last real taste of woman-to-woman intimacy until the kitchen coffee klatch, where toddlers bounced against us as we chatted. Now we are rediscovering friendship as we experienced it in our late teens and early twenties. And it is good. We wonder why it ever stopped. Finances got in the way, that's true, but the real obstacle was our own well-learned ethic: The man takes precedence. Being married and staying married pushed same-sex friendships aside. It's interesting to trace this ethic, this notion of woman as eternal competitor for the man. Hardly an atmosphere that fosters cordial woman-to-woman relationships.

Historically, women have found support, sympathy, and

understanding from other women. Their common experience
fostered a closeness quite different from the primarily economic ties to the men. Written documents of earlier centuries reveal strong bonds uniting female relatives and friends,
with common interests in domestic matters, the hazards of
pregnancy and childbirth, and the aching suspense of nursing
family members through illness. Because women's interests
were sharply divided from men's, each sex was more likely to
discuss matters of common interest with same-sex friends.

Also, there were more single women in those days. Wid-
ows and spinsters lived with the family, providing respite
from child care to the mother and support for each other.
This must have been helpful to mothers not only in practical
ways but as constant and present reminders that there was
more to life than children and husbands. We need that kind
of reminding even more today, because those of us who are
wives and mothers are often too preoccupied with the effect
of menopause on family members. We ignore our single
friends whose experience of menopause is different but no
less valid. We should be learning from each other.

Marriage has assumed more importance in this century
and, since the culture dictated that a married woman had
more status than a single woman, women began to view each
other as competitors for a scarce resource. Social life
marched two-by-two and "singles" were made to feel like
third thumbs.

When I ran my first Midlife Workshop for Women, the
energy generated by women sharing their life
experiences could have illuminated the room.
Throughout the workshop, women felt an intense closeness
and bonding with each other and kept asking, "How come
we've been so separated from each other all these
years? Why have we each felt so isolated?"
    Finally, someone said it: "Our men kept us apart. We
were so afraid of losing our men to other women that
we cut back on our female friendships!"

Women also looked for an ideal marriage relationship—a caring, supportive, understanding partner in whom to confide, on whom to rely, with whom to discuss and share everything. Very few marriages fulfill this ideal, and the high rates of divorce and separation during the last few decades are testimony to the disillusionment inherent in such an unrealistic expectation. But the majority of marriages endure and, because the illusion of an ideal marriage must be perpetuated, many married women continue to turn aside opportunities for friendship. Such women, by limiting their intimate friendships to one heterosexual relationship, are inviting spiritual anorexia—pointlessly starving themselves of friends.

Men often define a friend as someone to do things with. Women tend to define a friend as someone to talk to, to share feelings with. Women are more likely to recognize the connectedness of relationships; their decisions and actions take into account the effect on others, regardless of the absolute "right" or "wrong" of the situation. Where men see a hierarchy ("Who was in charge?" "Is that part of his job?"), women see a network ("Did everyone help out?" "How did she feel?"). For men, power and control take precedence; friendship must bow to rules that separate employee from employer, member from nonmember; women are more likely to overlook status differences where mutual interests are recognized.

Given these different ways of viewing the world, it is easier to understand why women are receptive to the idea of intimate friendship and so lost without it, and why men, although open to the idea of friendship *in principle*, will often forego it for the sake of a job, a title, the rules, or the team. What is hard to understand is female complicity in the "putdown" of women-only social situations. Women who fail to recognize the deep-seated male envy of female friendships may be lured into the trivialization of something that is important to everyone. Many women who once found support and sympathy in hastily convened kitchen meetings now attend more-formal business meetings. They find that, aside from the constant interruption of children, more problems were solved in those informal get-togethers than are solved by most highly organized committees.

No one should be without a friend. There are all sorts of opportunities in work (paid or volunteer), in educational or recreational settings, in social situations linked to work or club membership. Why, given all these opportunities, do some women still feel friendless? Part of it may be the low level of self-esteem that follows from being housebound. Some of it is sheer lack of experience in nurturing friendship. Some of it comes from a misplaced reticence about "personal matters."

> I learned very early in life that I couldn't trust my friends. Being a very sensitive child, it went pretty deep when I had been betrayed. Already a loner and middle child, it didn't take much for me to sort of abandon the human race and live a rather lonely life for many years. When I would occasionally long for a friend, of course there was nobody there. In recent years, I have stretched out my hand more and more (if you want a friend, you have to be a friend), but it is hard work for me. A few times when I have reached out to a person with whom I felt I had something in common, I was rejected. I blamed it all on myself but have since learned that I shouldn't. (I've always been hard on myself.) Maybe I was just trying too hard. I envy those who have cultivated true friendships but haven't given up hope yet of acquiring the same for me.

It is difficult to become intimate with a woman who avoids self-disclosure. It is impossible to complain about one's own husband (inconsiderate lout!) to a woman who admits no flaw in her own, to express outrage about one's children (ungrateful wretches!) to a woman who appears to have perfect offspring, to mutter about the ceaseless demands of an aging parent to a woman who is a Florence Nightingale. Perhaps such women feel that to admit to a problem would be to lower themselves in the eyes of others. Frankly, I find such attitudes a barrier to friendship. How wonderful to have a woman friend who makes no judgment calls, who allows you to unload all the anger, disappointment, and spite, and who is never surprised to find that, after all the anguish, you've forgiven and forgotten by the following day.

The female definition of friendship is percolating into the business world. As women break into higher ranks of management, customs of informal socializing on the job are not only being tolerated, but are being encouraged because they contribute to higher productivity and morale. Seminars run by women bring groups of business people together to talk about attitudes or habits that are impediments to personal or professional progress. These seminars are not promoted as teaching "feminine" skills, but that is precisely what is going on.

For many of us, female friendships grow sweeter as the years go by. Many of us have more time to spend with friends, to linger over a glass of wine, to visit for weekends, to meet for all-day shopping binges, or to spend a few days enjoying shared interests. This is one of the bonuses of menopause. The pain and the puzzlement can be shared with our women friends. Menopause gives us an opportunity to strengthen old friendships or to forge new ones—friendships that will stand us in good stead in the years to come when many of the men in our lives will have passed on.

Women who have chosen to remain single can teach us the value of friendship. Women without partners, whether through death or divorce, find that female friends provide a safety net, a web of caring to keep them from hitting bottom. Our friends are companions in new adventures, sounding boards as we embark on a new stage of life. They share a range of experience that is unique to woman.

Long-term Relationships

One evening after dinner, during my fifty-first year, I found myself pulling off my wedding ring and hurling it at my husband while I shrieked my intention of seeing a divorce lawyer. What had come over me? Too much wine, for one thing, and a great deal of emotional confusion. We didn't speak for the rest of that evening but we did climb into the same bed (every other bed being occupied that night). I woke up at two a.m., wondering whether I had finally lost my grip, and went downstairs to sit and think. Fortunately, my husband noticed my absence and came down to talk. We had had many, many emotional scenes in our twenty-seven years of marriage but we had *never* mentioned divorce before. And I had been the one to bring it up! I couldn't understand what was happening to us.

In successful long-term relationships, there is an unspoken agreement. When *he* is feeling dejected and discouraged, *she* will be upbeat and optimistic. When *she* is feeling worn-out and useless, *he* will tell her she's one in a million. Marriage consists, in large part, of cheering each other up.

Then along comes menopause and midlife. Frequently, both partners are consumed with their individual and very real problems, and the unspoken agreement goes out the window. At least that's my best guess at what happens.

Menopause often comes at a time when the husband is making a last-ditch effort to secure his place at work. The years just before retirement are the years that dictate the dollar value of his pension. They are also years when maintaining energy and dedication to the job may become more and more difficult. So the man is often under strain.

If there are adolescent children in the house, this adds to the tension. Even the best-behaved teenager knows how to manipulate parents to get his or her way, and that manipulation often creates a divisive atmosphere. One parent views the other as too lax or too strict. More havoc is caused by teenagers whose style of dress, taste in music, attitudes toward education or money (or both), become, implicitly or explicitly, threats to parental values. Such challenges to authority often arise at a time when Father is dealing with his own private insecurities, and when Mother is not feeling up to assuming her usual role of mediator.

Where the children are older and away from the house, there are other strains. Sometimes men are winding down their jobs just as their wives, newly liberated from domestic responsibilities, are gearing up. Many women in their late forties or early fifties bravely return to school or to the work force—or both—with the heady intention of now doing what *they* want to do. Women who have always been in the work force may find renewed energy for their jobs, as household chores take a backseat. The husband who has been looking forward to spending more time with his wife (now that the children are gone) may find that she is rarely there. She is wrapped up in new and exciting interests that he cannot or will not share.

Then there is the effect of menopause itself. It often brings on mood swings—emotional ups-and-downs that are difficult for both the woman and her husband to understand or contend with. There is something eerily reminiscent of adolescent emotionality in the yo-yo action of menopausal moods. But this is not the whole story. It seems to me that there has been too much focus on the mood swings of the menopausal woman and too little attention paid to the male half of the equation.

It is *assumed* that the woman is being difficult during menopause—and she may be. But many men continue to think of themselves as the sweet, good-tempered souls they were at age twenty-five or thirty. They forget about the invisible but unavoidable transfer of attitudes from work to home. If they have achieved any sort of authority on the job, that authority may also be exerted at home. The habits acquired when commanding others, when delegating chores, when minimizing complaints among subordinates, when problem solving, may get in the way of the ability to listen, to sympathize, and to learn. This may be even more true of the man who has not been as successful as he had hoped. His need for admiration and respect may get in the way of the intimacy that his wife had expected from long-term marriage.

One of the greatest threats to good marriage at midlife is the sense of vulnerability that many women feel. When they look at their husbands, they see people who are trudging through life at a steady pace, aging slowly but often attractively, looking more prosperous and more confident than ever. In our society, the media presents us with images of successful middle-aged men every day—in advertisements, in the news, in business appointments, in TV shows. The graying, slightly corpulent middle-aged man often achieves an air of distinction denied to him at a younger age. And why *shouldn't* he look distinguished? Heaven knows, he's worked hard enough for it!

Then we look at ourselves. We see signs of aging (thickened waist, graying hair, aching joints) that arrive too quickly to be properly assimilated. Positive role models are scarce. There are middle-aged women in show business who continue to look thirty-five, and a few women in public life who radiate confidence and competence. But it is hard to find a woman to emulate, an image to aim for. In a society that celebrates youth, we judge ourselves as second rate— physical well-being unpredictable, confidence sagging. It's hard to discuss this with a husband. Why point out to him how fat you're getting if he hasn't noticed? Why tell him how miserable you're feeling when you know (and he knows) that there isn't any *reason* for you to feel so unsure of yourself? How many husbands have terminated a conversation in exasperation: "Why not see a doctor?" How many wives have given up trying to make him understand?

For many years, when the kids were small, my husband often went to bed for a nap right after supper. By

the time he got up again, it was bedtime for the
children. On days he didn't nap, there was a meeting,
or a course to go to, or a workout at the local YMCA.
As a full-time homemaker, I cannot tell you how
disappointed, frustrated, and angry I was when I
didn't get the support I thought I needed—after having
already spent all day alone with the little ones.

I felt I just *had* to get involved in the community
in order to keep my sanity. Before long, I was into
various things which I very much enjoy but which keep
me away from home some evenings. Since I'm still a full-
time homemaker, with the kids at school and hardly
anybody to talk to during the day, my contacts with
these people in the evenings are my lifesavers. These
groups have—in the absence of any relatives in North
America—become my support system.

But now my husband is going through his own
"change of life" as well. He demands more time, attention,
ego-stroking, etc., and almost resents it when I'm out,
sometimes a few evenings in a row. He stays home
most evenings since he is feeling depressed and hasn't
much energy. Doesn't that sound familiar? Now and then
he says, "I don't seem to be too high on your list" or
"Do I have to make an appointment with you?" Not
only have I got nothing to spare right now in the way
of caregiving, but I also keep asking myself, "Where was
he when *I* needed *him?*" Besides, I feel I have to have
my own needs met for a change before I can be an
effective caregiver again.

Many of us had already learned to "keep a cap on it" during the few days prior to our monthly menstrual periods. At
"that time of the month," we could easily turn a minor skir-
mish into a full-scale war, so we learned (the hard way) to
grit our teeth and keep quiet. It seems to me that menopause
is often like a prolonged premenstrual period, but instead of
keeping a cap on it for two or three days, we may have to
keep mum for two or three years. This is not easy to do, and

we all forget our good intentions and blurt out hurtful criticisms now and then, but at least we're trying. And we're trying because we have a profound confidence in the viability—and durability—of the relationship.

It takes years to develop that kind of confidence: to know, at a gut level, that this is someone you want to spend your old age with, God willing. I know many women who don't feel that way. Some have decided to call it quits: the only common interest that had endured was the children. Others have decided to hang in: they are realists and recognize that they will never achieve the standard of living alone that they have become accustomed to as wives. I don't think men realize just how many women, smiling and compliant as they may appear, are living with these kinds of decisions.

I also know many women who have a great deal more in common with their husbands than they are willing to acknowledge. A divorced friend refers to her ex-husband as her "history"—as much a part of her, after more than twenty-five years of marriage, as part of her own body. She does not regret her decision to divorce, but it took the divorce to make her recognize this shared past. Another friend made a different decision. After living apart from her husband for almost two years, she swallowed her pride and decided to go back. They have no more in common than they had when she left, but they both appreciate each other more because of the separation. As this friend said, "Any habit is hard to break, and we had the habit of living together." Another friend is muddling through, as she says, by "reviving some of the customs of early married life." By this, she means being conscientiously *nice*—complimenting her husband when he does or says something positive, being more polite than usual and, in general, being as considerate as she was at the beginning of married life. Her hope is that the marriage will evolve, as it did once before, into a comfortable relationship.

There are a lot of marriages that exist in the space between commitment (contented or working-at-it) and hostility (veiled or open). Some are jeopardized by sexual matters: wives who find sexual desire absent after surgery or who can no longer experience orgasm as they once did, husbands who disguise their own faltering sex drive by blaming their partners. Some relationships are fraught with the fear of disappointing, haunted by one partner's sense of never quite reaching the promise implied so many years ago. Some couples are so busy looking at the *little* differences that they never stop to recognize large areas of their lives that offer mutual interest and delight. These are the marriages that could be enriched by a few sessions with a qualified marriage counselor.

The challenges and rigors of menopause will never be understood by a man. Expecting much more than tolerance and forbearance may be expecting too much. Marriage at midlife may not be too different from marriage at any other time— great, rotten, or somewhere in-between—but it may be all of these things within the span of one day. This may be a time to cherish what you've got, to put it on "hold" as best you can, and to promise yourself to be good to him when you're feeing better.

Male Menopause

For some time now I have felt that I, as well as my wife, am going through some bodily change. I feel on top of the world one day and just the opposite the next. I also don't have that "joie de vivre" that I was used to. What really concerns me is my sex drive, which at times just disappears. I am used to having a normal male sex drive and enjoy it very much; to suddenly have it evaporate for no reason is very hard to handle.

This letter conveys the essence of the so-called male menopause—the absence of sex drive. Actually, there is no such thing as "menopause" for the male, because menopause requires a monthly menstrual period, but the term has been freely borrowed to describe problems that sometimes bother midlife males—the absence of sexual desire and/or the inability to sustain an erection. Even when other symptoms are mentioned, these two assume paramount importance.

Male menopause is not the same thing as *midlife crisis*—a term that is applied mainly to men between forty and fifty. This age rarely marks the real midpoint of a man's life, but it assumes the earmarks of "crisis" because the fortieth year has assumed great significance for men in Western society. In Europe, the syndrome (if indeed it exists) is known as *andropause* and is receiving more and more attention from both social scientists and researchers.

Because the average adult male experiences a lengthy and very gradual reduction in the production of androgens, and particularly of testosterone, he is less likely to suffer from the kind of abrupt changes experienced by the average female at menopause. It seems likely, however, that *some* men (no one knows exactly how many) may be prone to sudden drops in hormone levels at midlife. The statistic that is frequently quoted is 15 percent, but it is not substantiated, and little or no attention is paid to other factors that might significantly affect testosterone levels (e.g., smoking, alcohol intake, and effects of medications).

Hormone levels are also influenced by stress. Many men in their late forties and early fifties are dealing with job-related tension—tension stemming from unrelenting effort, from pressure, from frustration, from apprehension, or from boredom and monotony. The tension may be compounded at home, particularly when there are adolescent children. The man may be consuming too much food and too much alcohol. He may be experiencing new and annoying infirmities—a sore back, bursitis, inflamed or enlarged prostate. Any combination of these symptoms could lead to *secondary* testicular failure, or the temporary inability to produce adequate amounts of testosterone. This leads directly to loss of sexual desire.

Sexual performance is so intricately tied to a man's self-image that emotion often supplants reason. For many men, it is not so much the reduction in sex drive that is threatening, but the loss of what is seen as "manhood." To avoid dealing with the problem, he finds excuses. He may work late and come home exhausted; he may stay up to watch late-night television, allowing his wife to get to sleep first; he may start arguments, which enable him to go to bed mad. In some cases, the wife may be held responsible for his inability to "turn on"—she is not inviting, or enticing, or aggressive, or compliant, or available enough. In extreme cases, he may turn to another (often much younger) woman to see if novelty can revive the desire he once took for granted.

The stress of feeling inadequate can lead to impotence, which is the inability to sustain an erection. This type of impotence will be considered secondary because there is no functional block to potency. One of the ways to determine if impotence is primary or secondary is to look at the man's capacity for erection when waking up in the morning, or during dream sleep. If he can have an erection at these times then impotence is considered secondary.

If impotence is believed to be due to primary testicular failure, tests will be ordered to measure testosterone and gonadotropin levels. (Just as women secrete small amounts of testosterone, men secrete small amounts of FSH, LH—and estrogen!) The tests are not always accurate, however. As we know from female physiology, very small variations in hormone levels can produce remarkable effects. Unless the tests demonstrate a clear physical malfunction, most doctors will assume it is *secondary testicular deficiency* resulting from stress.

Deficiencies in testosterone may be partly responsible for declining musculature, increased body fat, and thinner bones in aging men—and may also influence mood—but it is feared excess testosterone will increase the risks of heart attack. In addition, there is some reluctance to experiment with testosterone therapy because about 25 percent of men over the age of forty carry dormant cells which, if hormonally stimulated, could develop into prostate cancer. Because testosterone is customarily injected, provoking wild swings in testosterone levels, physicians who *do* administer testosterone are warned that the dosage should be carefully individualized. Some doctors look forward to the day when testosterone will be available through skin patches, similar to today's estrogen or nicotine patches.

Recently, research has looked to another hormone—human growth hormone (hGH)—which is used to treat children who stop growing, and which was also used in a controversial experiment that is alleged to have added muscle mass to twelve elderly men. Human growth hormone may be just as influential as other hormones (estrogen or testosterone) in delaying signs of age in both men and women. Secreted by the pituitary gland during normal childhood and adulthood, hGH levels begin to decline after age fifty. It is speculated that some changes usually attributed to normal aging might be caused by a deficiency of hGH.

Synthetic hGH was first marketed in 1985 and, although the primary recipients have thus far been children, the marketing of hGH as a rejuvenator for aging men is a distinct possibility. Cautious physicians have asked whether it is ethical to promote hGH therapy in cases where levels have not been demonstrated to be deficient. This hasn't stopped doctors from prescribing estrogen to premenopausal women, however, so it seems likely that aging men may soon be targeted in much the same way that women have been.

Dr. John McKinlay, epidemiologist and chief researcher of the Massachusetts Male Aging Study, reacts to the prospect of treating male menopause:

I don't believe in the male midlife crisis. But even though from my perspective there is no epidemiological, physiological, or clinical evidence for such a syndrome,

I think by the year 2000 the syndrome will exist. There's a very strong interest in treating aging men for a profit, just as there is for menopausal women.

The Empty Nest

According to the *Second Barnard Dictionary of New English*, the "empty nest syndrome" is a "form of depression supposedly common among women whose children have grown up and left home." The term was first used in a book published in 1952 but became common currency in the mid-1960s. The operative phrase is "supposedly common." For every woman suffering from empty nest syndrome, there are many others who feel guilty because they're so glad or relieved to have the children leave. The phrase is perpetuated, not by women, but by advertisers who push medication or new furniture as a cure for the temporary lull between stages of a woman's life.

The empty nest conjures up a picture of a woman alone in a house designed and furnished for a family. How applicable is this to women today? Not all women live in houses; not all are mothers with grown children; very few women spend their days at home. It assumes that women have neither the foresight nor the adaptability to take up new interests or activities as the children become more independent. It also assumes that the children have left for good.

Most of the women I hear from are not at all depressed by an empty nest. They find their ordered lives, their neater rooms, their freedom to come and go a welcome change. Many also think of themselves as "unnatural mothers," not realizing that all available research findings agree: There is a very welcome increase in satisfaction with life after the departure of the last child—less concern about the children, more activities with husband and/or friends, and increased marital happiness.

I can really relate to others who are saying good-bye
to their last child. Our youngest, who is now twenty-
three, has just moved out for the last time. He has
come home several times, but we have now told him that
this time he is on his own. We are hoping it will work
out since he is now sharing a home with his sister.
Guilt? None.

It is great to know you can cook for two and only
two will show up, and that there are times you can come
home to a tidy and empty house. I really enjoy being
able to go to bed at my early hour and have the house
quiet enough to sleep. My husband works shifts so I'm
often the only one home and I love it!

This is not to say that we don't experience strong feelings
as the children leave. The "launching" of the last child marks
the end of a period in our lives and forces us to acknowledge
the passing of time. I remember crying when my eldest
started first grade (I was expecting my fourth child at the
time!) and when I was folding away the baby clothes after
the last had outgrown them. Both events marked an end and
a beginning, which is why I cried. But there was no real
yearning to go back. And so it is for most women when the
last child leaves.

The real emptiness that many of us dread derives from
aspects of motherhood which are rarely discussed: the loss of
both intimacy and control. Motherhood involves enormous
power—a power that we acknowledge mostly in its negative
form as child abuse, but power nonetheless. With the departure of the children, many women lose a sense of power and
purpose that is denied them in any other sphere. This loss is
real and difficult to replace.

I believe I have a classic case of empty nest. I have five
children, the youngest now twenty-four and recently
out on her own. For the last four or five years, I've
been feeling guilty about actually wanting her to leave.

My marriage has never been the greatest, and I always
hoped that extended periods of time alone would help
the relationship between me and my husband.
Unfortunately, I find myself feeling more alone than ever.
My husband has never been a good communicator and
he continues to shut me out of his life. My problem
is one of conflicting emotions. On the one hand, I feel
relieved that my children are gone but I also feel enormous
guilt because I feel I may have pushed or prodded them
out of the house. Now that they're gone, I miss the
closeness and involvement in their daily lives,
something I never get from my husband.

The departure of the children creates a lull, and many of
us find ourselves off kilter as we grope toward new ways to
feel a sense of accomplishment. But this is a temporary lull.
Most of us can turn to friends, to work—volunteer or
paid—to a husband or lover to take up the slack.

A more common concern than empty nest, according to
my correspondents, is the child who leaves, returns, and
leaves again. Many women feel guilty that they don't miss
their children more after they've left. Many feel guiltier still
when the return of the child doesn't lift the heart, or lifts it
only for a day or two! And yet, in these days of mounting tu-
ition fees and extravagant apartment rentals, many young
adults *must* move home if they want to continue their education or get a leg up in the job market. And who is going to
turf them out?

A researcher in England investigated parents' feelings
about the empty nest. She found that mothers and fathers
felt very differently about the departure of a child, depending on the age of the child, where the child was going, the
personality of the child, and the relationship with the parent
or parents. This study highlights the complexity of a situation that has been simplistically exploited by the media.
Women who talk to other women recognize that each

situation—like each child—is unique, that the empty nest suggests much but describes very little.

The Sandwich Generation

Over the last few years, the term *sandwich generation* has become generally accepted as a way of describing midlife women and men who are required to deal, at the same time, with the needs of both older and younger generations—their parents and their children. More and more middle-aged women are experiencing the squeeze of the sandwich. Elaine Brody calls them "women in the middle," caught between the demands of the children (and often grandchildren) and the needs of aging parents. Many are also caught between seething resentment and bouts of self-imposed guilt.

Our parents can expect to live longer these days. This is not necessarily a result of improved medical care (although this does play a part), but simply because of better education leading to improved hygiene and nutrition. There are also *more* old people relative to the population as a whole. As families have become smaller and as immigration has slowed, we have seen a steady increase in the proportion of elderly in our society. Those over sixty-five now constitute 12 percent of the population; in only a few years, they will make up 15 percent. The aged are becoming more visible simply because there are more of them.

This has many effects. When the aged constitute a small proportion of the population, they are highly prized. They are the repositories of the oral history of a people, the witnesses to "the way we were." The child with a grandparent is special and is envied. As the aged population increases, veneration and respect for the individual yield to concern for and interest in the many. The study of all aspects of aging (gerontology) and the care of the aging (geriatrics) attract more interest and more tax dollars. Today researchers in the field no longer talk about the "old," but about the "young old" (aged fifty-five to seventy-five) and the "old-old" (aged seventy-five upward). The young-old are often the chief caretakers of the old-old.

One of the great ironies of the generation of women now dealing with menopause is that they often find themselves, after thirty years of hard work, better off than both their parents and their children. Most of us had expected to do better than our parents—this *is*, after all, the American dream—and many of us did. But the dream has faded for our children, who form part of the first generation to be denied a standard of living higher than that of their parents. This means that many of us are caught between the demands of a younger generation with extended dependency needs, and an older generation too proud to ask for help.

We may be forced to acquire new skills. As parents, we must adopt a tactful and neutral silence when our grown children make silly mistakes—the kind of mistake that *we* made when well out of the sight and sound of Mom and Dad. At the same time, we are required to muster diplomatic skills in order to intervene in the best interests of parents. For the sandwich generation, the problem is how to "be there" for children and for parents—to help out when needed and to stand aside when appropriate. It is normal and natural to resent the encroachment on one's time. It is also normal and natural to feel apprehension at the prospect of years of caregiving to parents, particularly when the caregiving of children must go on.

I feel like I am in a double-decker sandwich. I am, after twenty-five years of marriage, a single parent. I have a daughter twenty-two, and a son twenty, still living with me. I love them both dearly. I have been alone with them now for five years. They are adults, but, because they are living with me, they still demand a great deal of my time, directly or indirectly. They contribute financially, but emotionally, when you get three very strong-willed adults, there are bound to be waves from time to time.

Then there is my seventy-year-old mother who is not well, and who is unable to do much for herself. I do her errands and many other things. At first, I was foolishly running myself off my feet and found this very draining. I finally woke up to the realization that my mother, who had never worked out of the home, just did not realize the demands she was making on me. I am employed full-time and simply had to establish some priorities. Once she got to know when I would be coming over, that this would be regular and that she could count on it, there was no problem.

I don't think we should feel guilty if we put restrictions on our time. I think that what makes it difficult for the elderly is the uncertainty of their lives. Once they can rely on a regular routine (of visits, shopping, etc.), it is easier to cope.

Women reputed to be good managers can never rest on their laurels. The women who "cope" are the women who spring to mind when there is an unexpected need for someone to manage a crisis. Many events conspire to designate this "woman in the middle"—traditional attitudes about the roles and "innate" capabilities of women, experience with childhood crises, attention and sensitivity to family relationships. It is not justice that seeks her out, but rather her demonstrated ability to deal with one more family crisis.

This woman may still be the major caregiver for the children—those still at home and those who return. Chances are that she has always taken care of the weekly grocery shopping, the nightly dinner, the clean sheets, and the "pick-it-up-and-put-it-away." Women seem to be stuck with this role. And even though many of us work outside the home, we are married to men who take it for granted that men's work is more important than women's, and that wives are biologically programmed to take care of the needs and niceties of "family"—extending invitations, remembering birthdays, sending gifts, offering services. We may chafe at this particular role now (although it may have been a shared expectation 20 years ago) but, by fulfilling it, we are perpetuating it.

The "woman in the middle" recognizes herself. She knows, as do her brothers, sisters, and in-laws, that, when the time comes, she will be the one who is called upon. The story of the family where brothers and sisters spend equal amounts of time and effort amicably caring for aging parents must be a fairy tale. (Just like the one where other members of the family *don't* tell you what to do about the adult children still underfoot!)

Women feel guilty about resenting adult children and they feel guilty about resenting the demands of aging parents. Paul Ragan, an expert on aging, says that

> the most dominant and pervasive issue regarding inter-generational relationships is the subject of guilt. Often the adult offspring feel responsible for the general well-being of parents, [although they] frequently cannot improve their parents' general satisfaction with life.
>
> —*Aging Parents*, 1979

This issue of guilt is important because it is guilt that leads dutiful daughters to say, "They took care of me as a child; it is my turn to take care of them now." But taking care of a child is done with the expectation that the child will become more independent and more self-sufficient; this kind of expectation is *not* realistic in relation to aging parents.

What kinds of expectations *are* realistic? First of all, it may be *very* realistic to anticipate that you will do most of the worrying and most of the work. Sons tend to become caregivers only when they have no sisters and, even then, are more likely to call on their wives for "hands-on" help when dealing with their own parents. Sons may be called upon for financial advice and for menial tasks (lifting and carrying), but the women are almost always the primary caregivers. And the woman is typically a married, adult daughter (or daughter-in-law), a mother, and often a grand-mother.

> Last week, Mom phoned every night feeling terrible. I'd already taken time off (no pay) to take her to see two doctors and I had no car for two days. I finally phoned my brother and said, "You take Mom to the doctor's." "But, but ... I'm busy," etc., etc. Finally I said, "You do it!" And he did. Hooray for persistence.
>
> We are so used to being members of a generation where the woman does everything, it's hard to stop and say, "Excuse me, how about thinking about *me?*" We should get someone to shoulder it but that will never change for us.
>
> After Mom's second fall and hospitalization, I pulled over to the side of the road on the way home and had a good cry. I'm stressed but I can handle it. I have my man to complain to, my good friends, my workmates, and my daughters. Because I'm relating this situation to my own aging, I'm learning. The guilt never goes but I will myself through it and God gives me patience and comfort to understand and try to help. I might be in my mother's place soon and I'm thankful that I have two daughters who will care for me.

It is *not* realistic to expect that gratitude-for-services-rendered will smooth out rocky relations between the generations. If there is any kind of personality clash, it is likely to get worse, not better, as time goes on. Parents are always parents and they continue to feel and behave in parental ways. They are likely to stay the same, only more so, and their criticism or praise continues to have enormous influence on us, whether positive or negative. If they have no economic clout to wield, parents can still motivate us through flattery, gratitude, or guilt.

Nor is it realistic to expect that being surrounded by family will erase the void that the aged feel when continually confronted by the death of friends. Aging parents need friends. Family members, no matter how well intentioned, cannot substitute for the sense of well-being provided by friendship and common interests. You can help your aging parents to feel more comfortable, but you may not be able to change their general level of satisfaction with life.

It may be wise to examine your intentions, however honorable, and your motivation in assuming care of aging parents. Remind yourself that it is possible not to love someone and still care for him or her. Even if you feel genuine love for an aging parent, there will be times when you find it hard to like this person. Whether motivated by love, liking, duty, guilt, or a constantly-changing mixture of all of these, there will be times when you feel squeezed beyond recognition.

When parents feel that they can no longer cope with a young adult child who is not working, seems unable to find a job, is doing poorly at school, is planning to return home, seems unable to cope on his/her own, etc., most of us seek help. We turn to the resources that our tax dollars put in place. Academic advisers and trained counselors are available in high schools, colleges, and universities; they can tap into job retraining schemes, government bursaries, student loan plans, employment opportunities, or psychological services. If there is genuine conflict over goals set by you, your husband, or your adult child, then family counseling may be recommended. Most parents are likely to take advantage of such services, once they know about them, because it is for the child's ultimate benefit.

Unfortunately, many of us do not carry this attitude through when dealing with aging parents. Guilt gets in the way and we view the use of community resources as an abandonment of responsibility. We consider it a personal failure if we are unable to fulfill the needs of our parents, although this is as unrealistic as expecting to fulfill *all* the needs of our children, needs that are beyond our expertise and that cannot be foreseen.

Ideally, provision for care of aging family members should

take into account the opinions of the parent or parents. Even when aging parents deny the encroaching limitations of old age ("I'm fine, dear, don't worry about me!"), this is no reason to postpone planning for the future. At the very least, you can explore the facilities available in the community and plan accordingly. If your parent willingly participates in the discussion, so much the better.

Depending on such factors as income, time commitments, and geographical location, what responsibilities will be undertaken by other family members? What are your parents' financial resources, now and in the years to come? What kinds of alternative living arrangements might be acceptable to them, and what kinds of waiting lists do the "approved" facilities have? What kinds of community resources are available to help your parent(s) stay in their own home?

If a parent is seeing the doctor frequently, you may wish to find out if there is a Geriatric Screening Program available. This will permit a thorough and comprehensive examination without the necessity of making appointments with a number of specialists. The resulting report will give you and your parent(s) a clear idea of health status and may help to allay fears and/or lead to more constructive planning for the future.

Become familiar with the resources available in your parents' community—integrated homemaking care (cleaning and shopping services), Meals on Wheels, telephone checks, special medical alarms (easily tripped to elicit a return call and/or calls to a doctor, neighbor, nearby relative, or ambulance service), escort or transportation services, and help with home maintenance. You may be able to arrange for a public health nurse, podiatrist, or hair stylist to visit. (Care of the hair gets more difficult for women as they age, and care of the feet is particularly important if older people are to remain mobile and healthy.)

If you feel that a parent should not be left alone, you may be able to find sitting services. Some old age homes also offer "respite care"—short-term accommodation (from a few days to a few weeks) in a supervised setting so that the caregivers can have a weekend off or a vacation. It is wise to familiarize yourself with all of these services before you have to call on them.

Sometimes all the resources in the world cannot relieve the psychological stress of being responsible for family members. More and more community organizations are organizing support groups for caretakers of the aging. These groups may not be able to *change* the situation, but they can offer the opportunity to meet with others in the same situation, to air grievances, anxieties, guilt feelings, and to vent the anger that accumulates. It may also help you to deal with the frustration at your inability to "make it all go away," to make things better for your parent(s)—an inability that we may recognize intellectually but that is emotionally difficult to accept.

The "woman in the middle" lives between the stress of competing "guilts." Braced for the accusation that she has never been as good a mother as she had intended to be, she accuses herself of not being the loving and dutiful daughter that her parents deserve. The myth of the "good mother," coupled with the myth of the "good daughter," is powerful indeed.

REFERENCES AND RESOURCES

Angier, N. "Is There a Male Menopause? Jury Is Still Out," *NY Times*, May 20, 1992.

Blakeslee, S. "Men's Test Scores Linked to Hormone," *NY Times*, November 14, 1991.

Brody, E. W. et al. "Women's changing roles and help to elderly parents: Attitudes of three generations of women," *J. Geront.*, *38*(5), September 1983.

Brown, M. "Keeping marriage alive through middle age," in *Growing Older*, M. H. Huyck, ed. NY: Prentice-Hall, 1974.

Doering, C. H. et al. "A cycle of plasma testosterone in the human male," *J. Clin. & Endocrin. Metab.*, *40*, :492, 1975.

Donohugh, D. L. *The Middle Years.* NY: Berkeley, 1983.

Eichenbaum, L. and S. Orbach. *What do Women Want?* NY: Coward-McCann, 1983.

Horowitz, A. "Sons and daughters as caregivers to older parents: Differences in role performance and consequences," *The Gerontologist, 25*(6), December 1985.

Impotence: Current diagnosis and treatment. Education Office, The Geddings Osborn Sr. Foundation, 1246 Jones St., Augusta, GA 30901 (800-433-4215).

Lang, A. M. and E. M. Brody. "Characteristics of middle-aged daughters and help to their elderly mothers," *J. Marriage & the Fam., 45*(1), February 1983.

Lear, M. W. "Is there a male menopause?" *NY Times Magazine,* January 28, 1973.

Lehrman, S. "Human Growth Hormone: The fountain of youth?" *Harvard Health Letter, 17*(8), June 1992.

Levinson, D. J. et al. *The Seasons of a Man's Life.* NY: Knopf, 1978.

Lowenthal, M. F., M. Thurnher, and D. Chiriboga. *Four Stages of Life: A Comparative Study of Men and Women Facing Transitions.* San Francisco: Jossey-Bass, 1977.

McKinlay, J. B., C. Longcope, and A. Gray. "The questionable physiologic and epidemiologic basis for a male climacteric syndrome: preliminary results from the Massachusetts Male Aging Study," *Maturitas, 11:*103–115, 1989.

Moss, M. S. "The quality of relationships between elderly parents and their out-of-town children," *The Gerontologist, 25*(2), April 1985.

Notman, M. "Is there a male menopause?" *The Menopause Book,* L. Rose, ed. NY: Hawthorn Books, 1977.

Ragan, P. K., ed. *Aging Parents.* Berkeley, CA: Ethel Percy Andrus Gerontology Center, U. of Cal. Press, 1979.

Rosenthal, C. J. "Family supports in later life: Does ethnicity make a difference?" *The Gerontologist, 26*(1), February 1986.

Rubin, L. B. *Intimate Strangers: Men and Women Together.* NY: Harper & Row, 1983.

Rubin, L. B. *Just Friends: The Role of Friendship in Our Lives.* NY: Harper & Row, 1985.

Sanford, L. T. & M. E. Donovan. *Women and Self-Esteem.* NY: Anchor Press, 1984.

Sheehy, G. *Passages: Predictable Crises of Adult Life.* NY: Bantam, 1976.

10

Aging and Appearance

Aging is much more a social judgment than a biological eventuality. Far more extensive than the
hard sense of loss suffered during menopause ...
is the depression about aging, which may or may
not be set off by any real event in a woman's life.
—Susan Sontag, *Saturday Review,* 1972

Despite all the protestations (and reassurances) that menopause and middle age are two separate and separable events,
the lived experience of women fuses them. Menopause means
growing older, becoming invisible, losing one's power and
one's credibility. Our higher intellectual functions may insist,
"Not true! Not true!" But our experience—as eyes glance off
us, through us, by us—make menopause and aging indistin-
guishable.

A menopausal woman moves, quite suddenly and quite
unexpectedly, from a category of "secondary person" (status
based on sex) to a category of "nonperson" (status based on
age). This may sound extreme, but let me explain. As a
woman, one becomes accustomed to throwaway lines that
denigrate women: "She thinks like a man," "Just like a
woman!" and so many more. Some of us have learned to tune
into these kinds of remarks (many made quite unconsciously)
and to counter them. Those of us trained to examine and analyze social values may feel some satisfaction in alerting others to these entrenched and sexist attitudes and, in so doing,
limping toward the goal of equality between the sexes.

Then we run into ageism. It is difficult to combat social attitudes if you are neither heard nor seen. It is ageist when a sales clerk insists on serving everyone between the ages of twenty and forty before she condescends to help the sixty-year-old woman who got there first. It is ageist when doctors spend time explaining options to younger patients but then *tell* older patients what they must do. An aging person finds it more difficult to deal with ageism than sexism; he or she must attract attention in order to point it out. It is not aging that is difficult. Much of the pain comes from banging against solid, unseen, and unexpected ageist attitudes in this society.

Men appear to age at a fairly steady rate. The changes in hair color and texture, the alterations in girth and visual acuity, the gradual decrease in energy level are incremental and barely noticeable. There are not many men who look thirty-five when they're close to fifty, and those who do will go to some pains to look their real age. The appearance of youth for a man is a disadvantage in a society dominated by middle-aged men.

Both the process and prospect of aging are different for a woman. There are a great many women in their late forties who can easily pass for thirty-five. Because this knack of "not looking your age" is so admired, many women strive to look thirty-five for as long as possible. Some women just don't change much—a few laugh lines, a bit of gray at the temples—in the years from thirty-five to fifty. This resistance to the effects of aging, whether contrived or natural, sets the stage for what the French call "un coup de vieux"— aging overnight. Many women in their early fifties are plunged into despair because time suddenly catches up with them. At fifty-one and fifty-three, they finally look their age and, because they have looked thirty-five for so long, they appear to have aged fifteen years in five.

We live in a society that values women as decorative, sexual, and utilitarian. The first two are reserved for youth. Many of us find the third small comfort, although it helps us to be more understanding of the legions of middle-aged

women who become involved in committee work for religious
institutions or hospitals. The need to feel "useful" becomes
urgent when one is devalued in other ways. If the paid and
volunteer work of all women between fifty and sixty were
withdrawn for twenty-four hours, just imagine what would
happen!

The Need to Maintain Appearances

I feel that a valid role model for the middle-aged group
is lacking. How can you call Joan Collins a role model
when the principal reason she is lauded is because
she is *not* typical? I am one of those women who is fortunate
enough to look younger than her age. I find myself
frequently telling people how old I am so that I can
see the surprise register on their faces and get the
inevitable reassuring compliments about how I cannot
possibly be that old. And all this because it feels *good*
to get the reassurance that I don't look like what I
am.

I cannot feel good about myself when I am asking
others to help me deny that I am what I inescapably
am. I feel trapped by my looks. Trapped. When all
I want to do is give up and be me (whoever that is).

Many middle-aged women have no clear idea of what it
means to look one's age. Clothes, makeup, hair styles are all
modeled for us on much younger women. By showing us that
this is the way we are *supposed* to look, we are told, over
and over, that age is an enemy to be conquered. This is to
strengthen us for the battle, but it also serves to emphasize
the horror of aging—not only to women but to everyone else.
It is implied that any middle-aged woman could look like this
(model, actress) if only she *cared* enough. The truth is that
the role models shown to us—aging actresses or winners of

cosmetic manufacturers' contests—are individuals who, by dint of exercise or cosmetic surgery or genetics (or all three) do not look their age.

Exercise is beneficial. Each of us needs to have at least three hours of foot-pounding, arm-swinging exercise each week. This will enable our bones to remain strong, but this will not necessarily give us back the waistlines (and bust-lines) of our youth. A dogged regimen of aerobics implies re-wards, and Jane Fonda's empire of videotapes and walking tapes implicitly promise a Jane Fonda shape. But Jane Fonda is built like Henry Fonda, and *my* father (and proba-bly yours) wasn't built at all like Henry Fonda! We must ap-proach exercise in light of its real benefits and not in search of an impossible dream.

When I was taking my first course in word processing, I suddenly discovered that the little flashing light (the "cur-sor") would not move. I had been typing away quite merrily when suddenly I couldn't get any more letters to jump onto the screen. I hit keys at random (there are many extra keys on the computer keyboard) and, when nothing happened, I appealed to the teacher. She glanced quickly at the screen and said, "But you have a closed field." She then explained that, since I hadn't given prior instructions to the computer, it wouldn't accept any additional information. It was not in the right "mode."

I've always thought that this was a perfect analogy to my situation at the time. I was learning to use a computer with a view to perhaps launching a newsletter about menopause and midlife. I was feeling very discouraged about myself—both in terms of appearance and frame of mind. My mother was urging me to tint my hair, and I seemed to be moving into a larger dress size every few months. I had a clear idea of what kind of forty-ish woman I'd been and of the feisty old lady I intended to be, but I had absolutely no idea of what kind of person I'd be for the next fifteen years. I was so aware of my years that I lapsed into self-disparagement, re-ferring to myself as "a tired old woman" or "your old mother." (I winced when I heard myself, but I couldn't seem to stop it.) My field was "closed"—I couldn't find a realistic image of what I *could* be or what I *wanted* to be. I was suddenly confronting middle-age and I didn't like it.

From the letters I receive, I know that my own escalation from size 8 to size 12 is not unusual. I agonized about too-tight clothes for months, telling myself that it was because I had quit smoking and had nothing to do with menopause. (This was, after all, what most of the books said.) I think now that stopping smoking was responsible for my weight gain, but that the onset of menopause ensured that the weight stayed on. It took three years before I would look at myself, undressed, in a full-length mirror. Three years before I could begin to accept that the fat lady in the mirror was me.

Bodily Changes

There is always a time lag when there is a physical change: the self-image (which is a purely mental construct) and the real image (what others see) may not jibe and it takes time for these two images to match. This is true for those who lose a limb, those who lose weight, and those who gain. It takes time to get used to the new shape, and the adaptation period may not be particularly pleasant. Don't try to jam yourself into too-tight clothes; this just accentuates the weight gain. Pack away the clothes that don't fit (they may fit one day!) and start acquiring larger sizes. It helps if you have some idea of what you look like, so ask a trusted friend to point out women who resemble you in terms of height and overall shape. Chances are you will be pleasantly surprised to find you are not as gargantuan as you had imagined!

The problem I encountered with menopause was not so much the weight gain as the inability to shed those extra pounds. I weighed between 120 and 125 for most of my life and then, just as my periods started getting infrequent, I was up to 135! And it would *not* come off. I tried all the diets and I have finally accepted that this extra poundage is inevitable. I've gradually acquired a new wardrobe, have joined a fitness class, and am truly feeling good about myself. I even think that the slight padding on my face makes me look better (but I don't know if everyone else agrees).

Remember that the extra pounds are providing extra estrogen; that the precursor for estrone, the most important estrogen postmenopausally, is converted *in your fatty tissue;* and that this process will not only protect you from hot flashes, but will do so more effectively with time. Remind yourself that underweight women are more likely to suffer from osteoporosis. Better to gain weight at menopause than to suddenly lose weight.

How you move inside your body is often more of a giveaway than shape. If you're discouraged by your new size, concentrate on keeping your body firm and flexible. If you're already involved in doing regular exercise (as outlined in chapter 8), you will be able to gracefully accommodate the extra weight. If you walk with a spring in your step, consciously adopting an air of confidence, others will react to you more positively. When I gained weight, I was frequently told how *well* I looked. I mourn my "lost" figure, but the added pounds have taken away dark circles from under my eyes and added a certain roundness of cheek!

The Skin

If adolescence produces acne, then middle-age produces dry skin. Most of us can now indulge in bath oils, lotions, and moisturizers without having to lock them away from the reach of experimenting daughters. There are numerous products on the market: upscale products that feature models with flawless (and pore-less) skin; products aimed at "the wrinklies" (and marketed so successfully that our children buy us Oil of Olay for Christmas), and bins of products "on special" at the discount drugstore. The latter are probably as effective as any. Dermatologists recommend products containing petrolatum (Vaseline lotion, Nivea cream) or lanolin, and tell us to apply it while the skin is still damp. Rubbing Vaseline into the skin on your legs as you sit in a hot bath is as effective as using a high-priced body lotion. Buy soaps that have a minimal amount of perfume and detergent—clear soaps or Dove. Indulge yourself.

The skin changes in other ways. Many of us notice small red dots (cherry angiomas) appearing on the rib cage or stomach, or red threadlike marks (spider angiomas). Other marks appear such as small reddish or purplish marks or a tracery of small blood vessels under the skin. (When we see broken veins on the legs—our own or anyone else's—we tend to think of them as varicose veins. This is often wrong; many of these are broken veins that can be removed quite easily. Look for an expert, often an M.D., in sclerotherapy. The Yellow Pages may have a listing.)

One of the most hated skin changes is the appearance of liver spots (senile lentigos), which have nothing to do with the liver at all, but which show up on the backs of the hands, on the arms or on the face—and which darken after exposure to the sun. Some women also notice patches of scaly, dark skin appearing on the chest or back. These "moles" feel oily and thick to the touch and are just one kind of mole that may appear. Others are flat, dark "beauty spots" or pale "skin tags"—light-colored moles that hang away from the skin, usually at places that are constantly rubbed by bra straps or waistbands. All of these are normal. Tretinoin cream (Retin-A) is effective in fading liver spots: rub the cream onto the backs of the hands every night. The spots may take a few weeks to fade. Other types of undesirable spots can be removed by a dermatologist.

All my life I've looked on gray hair and liver spots as
signs of old age. These two superficial (when you think
about it) changes in appearance signified the "end
of youth" for me. I was really upset when I noticed liver
spots developing on the backs of my hands. I'd handled
the gray hair by regular sessions with the wash-in
hair coloring, but liver spots!! The only consolation
I have is that, after a summer of care-free sunning, a
couple of my friends started moaning about their liver
spots. Misery does love company.

As we age, our skin becomes more vulnerable to the ravages of the sun. Sunscreen is recommended for all ages, but
it is imperative for both youngsters and oldsters, and it's
wise to get in the habit of smoothing it on now. The skin
changes to worry about are the various forms of skin cancer.
Basal skin cancer starts with a pink, hairless, waxy-looking
growth, usually on the head or neck, and changes over time
to a cluster of shiny white pimples and then to a deep,
crusted sore. Squamous cell cancer starts as a small, hard,
red pimple, and then become a crusted sore that refuses to
heal—a sore with an irregular edge to it. Malignant melanoma (the cancer linked to imprudent and excessive exposure to the sun) starts as a slightly raised or bumpy, dark
brown, black, or blue area of skin with irregular edges, usually more than a quarter of an inch across, that changes in
color, shape, or size and which may feel itchy or sore. These
kinds of skin changes warrant an appointment with the doctor.

One of the most effective ways of encouraging healthy
skin is to do more exercise. Many of us have found that the
wintertime nuisance of dry, flaking skin on legs and arms can
be noticeably modified by regular workouts. If you can afford
it, regular body massage is both comforting and nourishing
to the skin. It's remarkable how many gobs of lotion can be
absorbed during a soothing massage.

The Face

Wrinkling is caused not by the outer layer of skin, but by changes in the connective tissue of the epidermis. With age, more and more of these connective fibers are produced and as you smile, frown, or grimace, the outer layer of skin creases to fit against the excess mass underneath. As you age, these creases get worn into the skin: the elasticity of youth is no longer there.

Premature wrinkles are caused by smoking (which produces wrinkles fanning out from the lips or corners of the eyes) and, most of all, by sunbathing (which dries the outer layer of skin prematurely). Cosmetic advertising would have us believe that the wrinkling process can be arrested, but it can't. Most cosmetics that claim to "prevent new wrinkles" contain a sunscreen, which is necessary in the sun but which may come too late to prevent wrinkles that are already there. Tretinoin creams may help, but this requires months of use and constant minor irritation (which plumps up the skin slightly and evens out the lines).

Almost all soaps dry the skin because they remove skin lipids (fats) and the skin's own moisturizing substances. There are all sorts of skin cleansers on the market but, if you need soap to feel clean, dermatologists recommend a mild soap followed by a moisturizer. Many suggest that the moisturizer be used on damp skin. Collagen-based cosmetics promise a restoration of the skin's *own* collagen (the protein that forms skin and bone), but the collagen actually comes from cows, and the molecules are too large to get past the skin's outermost layer. Collagen injections can temporarily plump up skin and smooth out wrinkles, but this is a different matter entirely. If there is no adverse reaction to collagen (some women are allergic to it), the benefits will last from six to twelve months. The injections must be done by an experienced dermatologist or cosmetic surgeon.

Estrogen is often discussed as a "cure" for wrinkling. Women who are small-boned and very fair often develop the kind of transparent skin, particularly on the back of the hands, that shows every vein. This often signals a serious depletion of collagen, not only in the underlying layers of skin but also in bone. These are the kinds of women most susceptible to osteoporosis and some forms of arthritis, and ET is often prescribed to halt the loss of collagen, or bone mass. Halting loss of collagen from the epidermis, the underlying layer of skin, does not affect the outermost layer, the dermis, which will still wrinkle.

The Hair

The appearance of gray hair is, in our society, a marker of age. We envy those who are prematurely gray (seeing it as unusual and special) and those who retain their natural hair color into old age. Most of us can expect to have 50 percent of the hair on our head go gray by the age of fifty. And at least 50 percent of fifty-year-old women will choose not to let this show, opting instead for at-home rinse-in "tints" or regular visits to the beauty salon for more permanent hair coloring.

There's no doubt that gray hair reinforces the image of middle-age. When I chose to go gray, the strongest argument I got against doing so was from my mother, who did not want an obviously middle-aged daughter! I decided to let nature take its course, however, because my hair was a natural auburn, which is almost impossible to reproduce, because it would take time and regular salon visits to keep it up, because the new gray hairs seemed softer and silkier than the natural red-brown "steel wool," and—most important of all—I was afraid I wouldn't know when to *stop* dying my hair. Whenever I went out, I would look for women who colored their hair: I saw too many who *should* have had gray hair but who were sporting false and/or harsh colors they had chosen years before. Who, I wondered, would come up to me and say, "Excuse me, my dear, but your hair color is so obviously false that you had better let your natural color show"? Also, I have to admit, my husband went gray *first!*

All this to illustrate that the decision about whether to go gray or not is highly individual. And the decision often has to be made before there are significant gray hairs. Somehow the natural color turns drab and lifeless just as the gray starts to creep in and, like it or not, you find yourself browsing the wash-in, nonperoxide products at the drugstore, looking for something to recapture the shine of healthy hair. Women who eat nutritious foods and exercise regularly may be less affected by this premenopausal drabness, but this is when most of us start seriously considering whether to use rinses or dyes.

Because gray hair is often finer, the gray tide may also bring an unwelcome thinning, from about 700 hairs per square centimeter of scalp to 500. Tinting the hair coats the hair shaft and adds body if the problem is a minor one. Often there is a family tendency to thinning hair, and often this happens in families where hair tends to be fine in texture to start with. Some postmenopausal women are affected by "male pattern baldness" and find the hair thinning either at the temples or at the crown of the head. This is assumed to be due to effects of adrenal hormones that are no longer being counteracted by ovarian hormones. Until recently, nothing much could be done about this. A product originally developed to alleviate high blood pressure is now being widely promoted. It is expensive, works for only 30 to 40 percent of those who try it and, even then, must continue to be rubbed on the scalp indefinitely to be effective. (If a woman suffers from patchy hair loss, this may be alopecia areata, a condition not linked to menopause.)

My hair, although fine, has never been a problem. As a matter of fact, it has always been very healthy and certainly plentiful. In the last six months, it has been falling out at an alarming rate. My husband seems to think I'm overreacting, but I figure I know my hair best and this is really scaring me! It's not only that it's falling out, it's coming out in patches. In other words, I'm losing hair in places like around my temples. I'm beginning to wonder if this problem is related to menopause.

Beauticians suggest that hair color should not mimic natural color; in most cases, the color chosen should be lighter. Ash blond may be too drab; deep brunette is probably too harsh. You might take a tip from the "punkers" and their hair of many colors: experiment with some of the new brush-in colors that disappear after one shampoo. If you are trying a nonperoxide rinse, choose a shade close to your natural color but warmer, and then gradually lighten the shade. Because one of these rinses lasts for a few weeks, the gradual change will probably not even be noticed. Keep your hair short—shoulder length at the longest—and use soft bangs or wisps of hair over the forehead and an uplift at the sides. Avoid backcombing, teasing, hair lacquer, or outdated "bouffant" styles. Hair mousse adds body without changing the color and can be combed into the hair each morning, if necessary. Another way of adding body is the body perm, which can be done at home, provided you use very large plastic rollers, larger than those supplied with the standard home permanent kit.

It's unsettling to have to deal with these kinds of changes. My hair, which had once been very wavy, became quite unmanageable for a few years, and I ended up having a series of curly perms because I was so awkward with a hair dryer or curling iron. Now that it is mostly gray, the wave has returned and I have gone back to finger combing it after a shampoo. In fact, in humid weather, my hair is wavier than it's been since I was a teenager. The analogy between menopause and adolescence holds, even for hair!

In addition to scalp hair, we must also deal with body and facial hair. Most of us notice a thinning of body hair—more and more infrequent shaving of the underarms, less need to shave the legs. On the other hand, the tweezers are needed more and more for stray chin hairs and, for women who tend to be dark and hairy ("hirsute") anyway, there may be the ominous shadow of a mustache. Of course, this whole idea of being hairless is a *learned* standard and quite silly when you think about it. There is no doubt that this society likes its women hairless to emphasize the childlike aspects of womanhood, whereas some societies find hairy women very sexy. Interesting how one can see this so plainly and yet feel compelled to banish all evidence of hair on the face, legs, and armpits!

Facial hairs seem to get worse during the menopause and then to ease up afterward. I noticed that the whiskers appeared on a cyclical basis even after I stopped menstruating. For one week of the month, I would feel them, get rid of them, and worry that my face would one day be covered in stubble. Now I find the whiskers appear only rarely. So don't panic if you are tweezing whiskers regularly. It may resolve itself in time.

Be aware, however, that certain drugs—some hypertensive medications, diuretics, antidepressants, and tranquilizers—encourage the growth of facial hair. Don't blame it all on menopause. Estrogen may diminish hair growth but should not be considered (or prescribed) for this reason alone. Spironolactone (Aldactone), an antiandrogen and diuretic, has occasionally been prescribed in low doses to reduce growth of heavy facial hair, although it takes some time for the effects to be seen. Medication should be a last resort; spironolactone may also inhibit sex drive and cause nausea, cramping, diarrhea, drowsiness, headaches, and other unpleasant side effects.

If facial hair is fair, tweezing may be the simplest solution; you will need a good magnifying mirror in a place with a strong light. If the hair is fine but dark, you may want to invest in facial bleach, which is readily available at a drugstore; the instructions are easy to follow. If the hair is dark and sturdy, you may want to try a new depilatory for facial hair, or remove it (or have it removed) with wax; there are

cold wax and hot wax methods. There are also special de-
vices available that pull out the offending hairs and that apparently lead to permanent hairlessness. Check your local
drugstore. Another permanent solution is electrolysis, which
kills individual follicles using an electric current. This has to
be done by a skilled operator and will require a number of
sessions.

Many malls have boutiques that sell cosmetics and also
offer free makeup sessions. I tried this once and received a
lot of useful tips. Because these malls are bathed in artificial
light, the amount of makeup applied may be too garish during daylight hours, but it gave me confidence in making myself up for swank evening events, where you want to look
your best and the lighting will tolerate a heavier hand. I
bought some of the small brushes in return for this free
makeup session: a fair trade, I thought. For women commit-
ted to the natural look, the use of makeup just takes up time
and money. But for those of us who like a touch of artifice,
self-enhancement becomes a challenge.

The Smile

More and more of us are looking to dentists to improve
our appearance. Some of this is involuntary as we all get
"longer in the tooth"—literally as well as figuratively—and
the periodontists get to work on our defective gums. Some
dental work is optional and cosmetic. It is no longer unusual
to see women of forty or fifty wearing braces on their teeth,
and orthodontists are attracting more middle-aged custom-
ers by offering sapphire braces, which are almost invisible.
Even more numerous are those who have their teeth bonded
to get rid of unsightly spots, the marks of old fillings, or to
minimize small chips or gaps.

Cosmetic Surgery

I resent those who look down their noses at the idea
of cosmetic surgery. It's no more artificial to extend
the youthful appearance of the face with a facelift than
it is to extend the elasticity of the vagina with an estrogen
cream. I suspect a moral judgment at work here: vanity
(self) is bad, sexual accessibility (other) is good. A
love of beauty is by no means the worst part of us.
I don't subscribe to the notion that lines are necessarily
an indication of character. Lines are an indication of lines.

Not all women are interested in having cosmetic surgery;
not all of us are candidates, because a number of medical conditions dictate against it, including hypertension, heart disease, diabetes, and not all of us can afford it. When we think
of cosmetic surgery, facelifts immediately come to mind. But
more and more women are turning to cosmetic surgery for a
body lift.

Body contouring, as it's euphemistically known, is not a
substitute for dieting or exercise. In fact, it is not recommended for those whose weight tends to fluctuate. The ideal
candidate for this operation has localized areas of excessive
fat, an otherwise normal and fairly stable body weight, and
good skin elasticity. Where skin has lost this elasticity (a natural effect of aging), a complementary operation to remove
excess skin (an abdominoplasty, or tummy tuck) may be
performed—either at the same time or some weeks later.

Fat suction (also known as suction curettage, lipectomy,
or lypolysis) is done under either local or general anesthetic,
depending on the extent and duration of surgery. Fat suction
of the abdomen requires three incisions, one at each end of
the pubic crease and another at the navel. For pads of fat in
places such as under the breasts or on the sides of the waist,
additional incisions may be required. A long-handled looped
instrument is inserted into each incision and moved around
to break up the cells, then a miniature wand (similar to the

extension on a vacuum cleaner but much smaller, of course) is inserted and moved about under the top layer of skin to suck out the fat.

After the fat has been vacuumed off, drains may be inserted and incisions closed with a suture. The drains are removed after twenty-four to forty-eight hours, but the incisions are left open to allow for additional drainage. The patient is allowed to walk the evening after the surgery and shower forty-eight hours after the operation. The hospital or clinic stay will be from two to five days, with pressure dressings required for three weeks and, for older patients, an abdominal girdle for a week or two after that. Patients can usually resume normal activity in a week or ten days, and heavy exercise in three to four weeks. A change is noticeable within three weeks of the operation but, because damaged cells will continue to be sloughed off for some time, it may take a month or two for the full benefits to show.

Severe bruising follows from the operation, but the extent and duration of the bruises will depend on age, coloring, and other factors. There is often a "rippling" effect on the skin—in other words, the skin does not necessarily go back to the smooth contours of youth. If the rippling is still unacceptable a month or two after the operation, a second procedure may be required. Potential side effects are necrosis (death of clumps of cells), which may require additional surgery, and unexpected and disfiguring scars.

Fat suction may seem like an easy solution to abdominal padding, but there are disadvantages at menopause. The ethical plastic surgeon wants to operate on a person whose body weight is relatively stable and who will, therefore, derive a long-term benefit. For many menopausal women, the change in shape (whether or not it involves a weight change) is only part of the picture. Often there are fluctuations in energy levels or temporary feelings of anxiety, panic, or even depression. In such a state of flux, the trauma of anesthesia combined with the shock of surgery may merely *add* to the physiological strain, putting *more* stress on a body already under siege. A well-known New York cosmetic surgeon has commented that such operations "buy time" for the woman not prepared to deal with the reality of aging. My own feeling is that it is better to confront aging and then, when you're feeling good about yourself, to reward yourself with smoother eyebrows or a flatter tummy.

It is estimated that about 10 percent of cosmetic surgeries entail some unexpected and negative outcome. Surgeons are responsible for the conduct of the surgical procedure, but there is no guarantee of satisfactory results. For this reason, any woman seeking surgical treatment should be very wary. Make sure you are dealing with a board-certified surgeon because, in this country, any licensed physician can legally perform any kind of surgery. To be board-certified, the physician must complete a two- to five-year residency in a surgical specialty and pass the qualifying examinations.

No matter what kind of operation you choose, you should get a referral or recommendation from a family physician or from former patients who have had the same operation. If you are contemplating body contouring, check with the American Society of Plastic & Reconstructive Surgeons (800-635-0635). This organization, or the American Academy of Cosmetic Surgery (800-221-9808) may be able to provide names of doctors in your area. If you are contemplating facial surgery, you might want to contact the American Academy of Facial, Plastic & Reconstructive Surgery (800-332-FACE). If your chosen doctor is affiliated with a hospital, you will know that he or she has also had to conform to certain hospital standards in order to use their facilities. If the doctor practices in a private clinic, you may want to check to see if he or she *did*, at one time, have hospital privileges. If the doctor has a university appointment, or is with a teaching hospital, this is usually considered a plus.

When you see the doctor, ask how many similar procedures he or she has performed and when. If the doctor is evasive ("Don't you worry about that; I know my business"), excuse yourself. Any surgeon should be willing to answer this question frankly and honestly. If you don't know anyone who has undergone the same procedure, ask to see photographic results of other operations. If former patients are willing to be contacted, ask to get in touch with them. The more information you have, the better.

Before you start your investigations you should be aware that, because the surgery is for cosmetic purposes, it will not be covered by health insurance and thus can be very expensive. The exception is breast reduction, which may be covered.

Last spring I had a facelift. This was not common knowledge, but my close friends knew about it and a couple of them came down hard on me for deciding to go ahead with it. It's funny because, although I had severe misgivings about "postponing" the aging process, I feel I am benefiting from the operation.

As women, we are continually reminded of the importance of our looks. It seems odd, then, that after years of emphasis on makeup and clothes, we're chided for trying to improve ourselves when we get to fifty or fifty-five. Granted it's a drastic and costly step, but I found it made a difference in my attitude to myself and, I think, in the attitude of my students toward me. I guess I look more "with it" now so they seem to pay more attention to what I have to say. Or maybe I'm just imagining it!

The ultimate response to the specter of aging is, of course, the facelift. This procedure (rhytidectomy) requires a hospital or clinic stay of from one to three days, another week of isolation, and three more weeks before the swelling disappears completely. The effects last from five to eight years. An incision is made in the scalp behind the hairline at the temple, descending to the front of the ear and back up behind the ear. If neck tissue is to be removed, the incision will extend downward from behind the ear and into the neck.

Possible complications are hematomas (swellings containing blood), which occur in from 10 to 15 percent of cases and which must be drained. In addition, it is impossible to predict changes in skin pigmentation or the kind of scarring that may result. In rare cases, injury may be caused to a facial nerve.

Chemical face peeling is a procedure that burns off the top layer of skin and that is often used to remove fine wrinkles around the mouth and eyes. It takes from four to twelve weeks for the skin to appear normal, and you will have to stay out of the sun for a full year. Possible long-term effects are scarring or changes in skin coloring. Dermabrasion is often mentioned as an alternative to chemical face peeling, but it's more useful for acne scars than for wrinkles.

For pouches under the eyes or hooded eyelids, some women resort to the eyelift or blepharoplasty. The operation for the lower eyelid is more difficult and, if done improperly, may prevent the eye from closing properly. Eye surgery usually involves an overnight stay at a hospital or clinic and can be done under local anesthesia. The patient must keep a compress on the eyes for at least ten hours, often longer, and this is usually the part of the procedure most difficult to tolerate. It takes about ten days to recover and two months before the final effect is achieved.

For bags under the eyes that are primarily composed of fat, a newer technique uses an electrically heated needle to vaporize the fat. Done under local anesthesia, this procedure takes about thirty minutes and heals in about a week. Plastic surgeons can use this same procedure to remove pads of fat under the chin. A nonsurgical solution to hooded eyelids is a piece of medical adhesive that is specially designed to hold up the kind of eyelids that fold right down to, or past, the eyelashes. This product can be used daily.

Makeup and Fashion

Whether or not you choose to spend money and time on cosmetic surgery, you still want to look your best. When you start to notice a loss of luster or color in your hair (whether tinted or not), you will also notice changes in skin color. If you continue to use the same makeup colors and techniques at forty-five as you used at thirty-five, you are probably doing yourself a disservice. The experts say that, as you age, you should conscientiously try to be more deft, more subtle with makeup, matching foundation carefully to skin color and abandoning rouge for a carefully dusted-on contouring powder.

Soft pencil can be used under the eye and along the upper lid, but it should be softened or smudged to avoid a hard line. Reddish-brown or pinkish-brown eye shadow is more natural than turquoise or blue. If you wear glasses, you can use more eye makeup, because glasses soften the effect.

For cracked or chapped lips, use a lip balm, wipe to remove dead skin, and use a lip primer to prevent "bleeding" of lipstick into lip creases. These primers are expensive but they last a long time. A lip pencil will also help to keep the lipstick inside the lines. Also, as small wrinkles appear around the mouth, any lipline that does not follow the natural lipline appears more and more false. Softer lipstick shades are more flattering to the midlife woman; they put less emphasis on the mouth and more attention is drawn toward the wise and worldly eyes!

We are fortunate in that fashion options are so wide these days. Despite the announcements that "waists are nipped" or "skirts are shorter," we can pick and choose in a way not available to midlife women twenty or thirty years ago. Coping with bodily changes means more than buying the same old thing but in a larger size. A skirt hangs differently over a budding tummy, and the waistband cuts during a temporary episode of "bloat." It seems strange to feel pantyhose, panties, and skirts all clinging to different parts of one's middle; the waist seems to be everywhere and nowhere.

Not long ago, I read the remark of a fashion expert: "Middle-aged women will love the shorter skirts because the legs are the last to go." Despite the anger I felt at this woman's patronizing remark, I had to admit that there was a grain of truth. Few of us worry about gaining weight on our legs. There is a tendency for weight to accumulate around the waist, on the diaphragm, across the back—a different story from the heavy hips and thighs that are common problem areas at younger ages.

Midlife women need elasticized waistbands, pleats that are stitched down to the hip or that fall from a yoke, big tops that sit easily on the hips or skim down to the old "three-quarter" length. We need bright touches of color to cheer us up and to flatter our changing hair and skin color. How many of us tune into reruns of *The Golden Girls*, not for the story line, but to get ideas for suitable clothes?

Women are motivated to seek adjustments to their appearance for a number of reasons. Some are touched by the "now-or-never" syndrome—the same syndrome that incites a midlife woman to leave a marriage or to start a business. These women will go in search of the straight teeth, the firm chin, the wide-open eyes that they have fantasized about for years. Other women find that their physical appearance just does not *fit* with their personalities; for them, worn wrappings do not fairly represent the up-to-date contents.

These may not be the women you think of in connection with cosmetic surgery, but they are as much a part of the picture as the common stereotype of the woman frightened of aging, the woman who blindly seeks help from a surgeon rather than confronting her own nightmares. We rarely notice the surgical enhancement of the stable woman; what we remark on are the aging women with the incongruously young faces. The tragedy of such women is that their movements and attitudes are so antiquated, so aging, that the facelifts are merely grotesque.

Because the aged are devalued in this society, most of us find any evidence of aging unwelcome. In one study of middle-agers, more than one-third voluntarily cited changes in physical appearance as a concern. There is no doubt that, for many women, menopause brings many changes; it's not easy to cope with a new shape and a new image. But, if we're realistic about it, we will acknowledge that it is not being fifty that bothers us, but rather the prospect of being viewed as "old." If menopause is on the doorstep of old age, then we have to confront our fear of aging.

I'm very conscious of getting older. I don't really want to be old. I'd like to put the clock back to about forty and stop there because, although I enjoyed the children when they were little, at forty I was enjoying my job. I was on top of the world. I was full of bounce. . . . I'm a bit afraid now that I'm over fifty. I can see sixty coming and I really feel that that is very old. . . .

I can see retirement and, although my husband says we'll go around the world and all sorts of things, my fear is that by the time we're old enough to do these things, we won't be young enough to enjoy them. I'm afraid that I will deteriorate very quickly when I get older.

I'm afraid that tiredness is going to stay with me and, in fact, increase. That really frightens me. I can't bear to think of not being well. I don't mind being old so long as I'm well.

The Need to Confront Our Own Aging

For many of us, growing old means not being needed. We all want a little niche where our presence will be noted, appreciated and, in our absence, missed. Many women's lives are unbalanced from being needed too much for too long, and then suddenly needed too little. One friend who has been forced to move away from her grown children and back to the place where her husband wants to grow old, says it has put her "off balance." No wonder. It requires enormous resilience to cope with a social worth that can so quickly redefine one from "essential" to "nonessential."

Years ago, I was pushing our baby carriage toward the house. In the carriage was my new baby girl and her seventeen-month-old brother. On a little chair fitted over the carriage sat my eldest, not quite three. Rain was threatening and I was about to break into a trot when a little old lady stopped me, peered into the carriage, and said sweetly, "Ah, my dear, these are the best years of your life!" I remember the rage I felt that anyone should label these the "best" years of my life—years of constant fatigue and incredible self-doubt. What a price to pay for being needed! (It made for a nice irony when, twenty-five years later, I was filmed for a National Film Board production titled, *The Best Time of My Life: Portraits of Women in Midlife.*) Is it possible to designate any years as the "best"?

There are different ways of being needed. We may fulfill basic needs (food, clothing, shelter, love) or we may fulfill secondary needs (advice, friendship, affection, touching). If we spend a large part of our lives dispensing love with hot meals and clean clothes, we sometimes confuse them. We fear that when we are no longer needed to cook, shop and "do" for others, we will no longer be needed. But we are needed to love them, as we have always done. It is normal to feel a sense of loss when one role ends and another has yet to begin. The gap created may leave us "off balance" but not, I hope, too timid to reach out to others who need us—who need our advice, our friendship, our touch. We *can* make a place for ourselves at this age, as at any age. The gap closes.

Closely allied to the fear of not being needed is the fear of having no central objective or purpose to one's life. Menopause often coincides with other major events in a woman's life—the end of "active" mothering, the awarding of the twenty-five-year pin to the faithful employee, the sudden and saddening loss of a parent or spouse, the growing awareness that one may be destined to spend old age alone. Those of us who thought that we would feel great satisfaction when we surveyed our grown children find, instead, that it is all a blur. These young adults, fine as they are, seem to have appeared out of nowhere. Now married, separated, divorced, or widowed, we have to look for new means to achieve satisfaction, the sense of a job well done.

At the same time, there is often a sense of being very *tired*, too tired to undertake anything new or different. You may just want to be left alone. I believe that this fatigue has its reasons. The body is adapting to a new internal rhythm and you need time to rest and to think. Middle age allows time for the reactivation of old dreams, the challenges of new learning, the tentative acquisition of new skills. When your energy comes flowing back—as it will—you will have found a cause, an activity, a source of satisfaction that will give meaning to what you do in the next major stage in your life.

It is during this pause, the real gift of middle age, that we should take time to examine our fears of aging. Today, confronted with new facts about the patterns and prevalence of Alzheimer's disease, we find ourselves nervously joking about menopausal forgetfulness, dying brain cells, premature senility, but there is often a deadly serious edge to our humor. We fumble for names, lose objects that turn up in the most mysterious places, notice that every stranger we meet looks like someone else (are we really that old?), and remember arcane bits of information from childhood. Psychologists tell us that this is a different kind of memory, no better and no worse than the memory of youth. They also tell us that women (who are usually held responsible for remembering the trivia of everyday life) worry far more about loss of memory than do men, although the changes in memory are similar. Victims of Alzheimer's rarely worry about loss of memory, because one of the symptoms is an inability to realize that they have forgotten something.

Like the fear of forgetting, the fear of becoming dependent is often expressed in black humor—for instance, the T-shirts and bumper stickers sold in Florida: "Avenge yourself. Live long enough to be a burden to your children." No one wants to be dependent, and this is one of the greatest fears of aging. Most of us know old people so haunted by this fear that it can never be spoken. There are no discussions, no contingency plans.

If this fear dogs you, take this time to examine your economic future. The government listings in the telephone book can guide you to information about pension plans. If you have a pension plan at work, you should be getting regular statements of your pension status. You can discuss this with your local bank manager and augment it, if possible, with savings. If you are dependent on your husband's pension, make sure you know what the provisions are. The American Association of Retired Persons (AARP) can provide valuable information about how to plan for old age.

There are, of course, other forms of dependence aside from financial dependence. Many of us are frightened by the prospect of having to depend on others for routine help—shopping, driving, fixing things around the house. In our determination to take care of ourselves, we often forget the joy that comes from giving. There is a time to give and a time to allow others to give to us. In the meantime, we can do our best to assure our independence by paying assiduous attention to healthy living. By taking good care of ourselves now, we may ease the minds of our children and lighten the burden of those who will have to take care of us in our old age.

Middle age gives us a marvelous opportunity to prepare for being old. We have time to dream about, and to plan for, the future. Even if we are feeling under strain right now, we can anticipate years of good health and renewed energy that will enable us to get involved in new projects and new causes. We have the mental acuity, flexibility, and experience to deal with shifting relationships and with generations both older and younger. We have the freedom to adopt new eating patterns or new activities that may very well keep us healthy for years to come.

I am often asked about the *good* things about menopause. It isn't hard to find them.

First is the sense of freedom. We are free to experiment with new kinds of foods, new kinds of activities. We are free from the necessity of stocking sanitary pads or tampons or of scheduling events around the ups-and-downs of the menstrual cycle. We are free to strike up a conversation with a stranger in a bus, or on a street corner, without being thought of as forward or seductive. We are free from the compulsion to work toward thinner thighs, or a twenty-four-inch waistline, or the perfect fingernails that we once longed for, and we are free to realize that it was a pretty silly ambition anyway! We are free to adopt our own standards of dress and decorum, guided more by good sense and comfort than by, "What will people think?"

Then there is the sense of getting another chance. Because menopause often brings us up short, psychologically and physiologically, it gives us a rare opportunity to evaluate where we are coming from and where we want to go. Because of this enforced disruption, many of us have found that we were continuing to do things that we didn't really enjoy. It was part of the routine and we hadn't stopped to think about it. Every day, middle-aged women are giving up cooking to take up woodworking; are boycotting movies in order to save for trips to faraway places; are enrolling for piano lessons, or computer science, or philosophy courses. Women are making changes that are not perhaps significant in themselves, but that allow for the expression of very personal interests—interests that sometimes have been lurking beneath the surface for years.

Finally, menopause gives women an opportunity to make friends. Because so little is known about the causes and effects of menopause, the only real understanding of it comes from other women. Menopause provides the perfect excuse to reach out to other women—to revive old friendships and to forge new ones. We know that the nourishment of friendship is a vital ingredient to a happy old age. We know that women are much more likely to survive into old age than are men. Thanks to menopause, we can enrich our lives now and carry these riches with us into an active and satisfying future.

REFERENCES AND RESOURCES

American Academy of Facial Plastic & Reconstructive Surgery: Hotline (800-332-FACE; in DC, 202-842-4500).

American Association of Retired Persons, Box 199, Long Beach, CA 90801 (Membership fees are $10/one year or $24/3 years).

American Society of Plastic & Reconstructive Surgeons, 233 N. Michigan Ave., Chicago, IL 60601 (800-635-0635).

Baruch, G. and J. Brooks-Gunn, eds. *Women in Midlife.* NY: Plenum Press, 1984.

Beeson, W. H. and E. G. McCullough. *Aesthetic Surgery of the Aging Face.* St. Louis: Mosby, 1986.

Berkun, C. S. "Changing appearance for women in the mid-years of life: Trauma?" *Older Women: Issues and Prospects.* E. Markson, ed. Lexington, MA: Lexington Books, 1983.

Chernin, K. *The Obsession: Reflections on the Tyranny of Slenderness.* NY: Harper & Row, 1981.

Cosmetic Surgery Information Service, American Academy of Cosmetic Surgery (800-221-9808).

Fairhurst, E. "Mutton Dressed as Lamb: The Social Construction of Aging." Paper presented at the 1st International Conference on The Future of Adult Life, Noordwijkerhout, The Netherlands, April 1987.

Le Guin, U. K. "On Menopause: The Space Crone," *Medical SelfCare,* Winter 1981.

Melamed, E. *Mirror, Mirror: The Terror of Not Being Young.* NY: Linden Press, 1983.

National Institute on Aging, Information Center, 2209 Distribution Circle, Silver Springs, MD 20910.

Rees, T. D. and D. Wood-Smith. *Cosmetic Facial Surgery.* Philadelphia: Saunders, 1973.

Rubin, L. B. *Women of a Certain Age: The Midlife Search for Self.* NY: Harper & Row, 1979.

Sontag, S. "The Double Standard of Aging," *Saturday Review.* 182–190, Sept. 23, 1972.

Stehlin, D. "Erasing Wrinkles: Easier Said than Done," *FDA Consumer,* July/August 1987.

Teimourian, B. *Suction Lipectomy and Body Contouring.* St. Louis: Mosby, 1987.

Appendix:
Where to Find or Get Help

Today there are many more resources available for the menopausal woman than there were ten or even five years ago. The major and most useful resource is simply more general information on the subject of menopause in the form of books, booklets, newspaper and magazine articles, films, and radio and television programs. Many organizations also offer information on particular aspects of menopause. Many of these references and resources are listed at the end of each chapter or in the Bibliography.

When you read one book, you may think you have found all that you need to know. If you read two, you are likely to find such diametrically opposed points of view that you will be compelled to read a third! If your local public or school library does not have a book you are looking for, it is worth making a request. Menopause is a subject of interest to growing numbers of people, and most libraries are willing to order a book at your request.

In addition, many organizations produce printed materials dealing with the more general aspects of menopause, or with specific problems that may be more troublesome to you (migraines, hysterectomies, etc.) Much of this material is free or available at low cost. You can obtain more information by writing to or calling the particular organization, or you can contact a local woman's health organization or woman's center. They should be glad to help you find resources to fit your needs.

Menopause Clinics

Some hospitals, particularly teaching hospitals, have menopause clinics. When a woman calls me with a list of debilitating complaints and nowhere to go, I may suggest that she contact a local menopause clinic. It is not advice that I give lightly.

First of all, most women will not need the medical support of a clinic if they are seeing a doctor regularly. What they *may* need is a more understanding doctor, but the time to shop for a good doctor is before you need one. If you are not satisfied with your present doctor and you are approaching menopause, it is a good idea to ask around and get the names of three likely doctors, and then make an appointment to see each in turn. If you are not experiencing any problems associated with menopause, you probably won't need to consult a doctor, and if you have a good doctor, you may not need a menopause clinic.

My basic quarrel with the menopause clinic is the confusion about its function. The main goal of a menopause clinic is *understood* by the general public to be the welfare and well-being of menopausal women. However, the primary goal of many newly founded menopause clinics is to provide data for menopausal research; helping women is secondary. Menopause clinics are usually subsidized (and supplied) by pharmaceutical companies. This means that, whether you know it or not, the "solutions" found for you may fall within the restricted purpose of the current research study or studies.

Most of these clinics have long waiting lists and, when you finally get an appointment, you may find that you are given a certain type of drug in order that the doctor may report on its effectiveness, or you may be told that you are to take a certain drug when, in fact, you have been given a placebo—a substance that looks like the product being tested but that has no effects.

There is nothing inherently wrong in this. Because of the low priority given to funding of research into women's health—a situation that is changing, I am glad to say—most hospitals *must* accept funding (and drugs) in order to continue their work. However, there is a fundamental difference between a menopause clinic and a menopause research project, and I believe this should be made clear to the women who attend. Many women go to a menopause clinic expecting individualized attention to their particular complaints, answers to their questions, and information about a range of possible treatments. This is an understandable expectation, given that their own doctors may be unprepared to deal with concerns about menopause. What these women may get instead is routine treatment as specified by the particular study underway—perhaps a general medical checkup, a short meeting with a psychologist, a short meeting with a dietitian, medication, and another appointment.

If medication is prescribed (or administered), this, too, will conform to whatever is being studied in this particular project. It may be an estrogen-androgen product, a combination estrogen-progestin patch, estrogen gel to rub on the abdomen, an estrogen tablet, a progestin tablet, or a placebo masquerading as any of these. The research study will be geared toward a particular type of drug, so that treatment varies from clinic to clinic, because the study (and the particular drug involved) will be tied to the funding of one pharmaceutical company. In other words, the menopause clinic's solution to most menopausal ailments will be a hormone preparation.

Some clinics do get involved in studies dealing with sexuality, or with psychological symptoms. If a woman is aware of the current research underway, she will find it easier to decide whether or not to participate and, if she does, to understand and cooperate with the process. She may also wish to ask for copies of the completed research papers.

Not all menopause clinics are this narrow,* although I know of one that threw open its doors, welcomed patients until the study results were in, and then promptly closed. Potential patients were told that it had been too popular, but the truth was that the research funds dried up.

There may be a menopause clinic available in your community that does *not* operate in this manner. Your best bet is to inquire about sources of funding and medication provided by the clinic before you enroll.

Menopause Seminars

Hospitals, women's health centers, and service organizations (often in conjunction with hospitals) occasionally present one-time menopause seminars or information sessions. These sessions, however they are labeled, usually take place in a medium to large hall (often a hospital or university auditorium) and permit very limited questions and answers from the floor. Most will feature medical experts, usually a doctor or doctors (sometimes a psychiatrist), occasionally a physiotherapist, and/or dietitian. These types of sessions often appeal to very busy women who want a quick, one-shot dose of information.

The basic problem with these kinds of sessions is that they often ignore the great diversity of opinion within the

*Pioneer and comprehensive menopause clinics exist in San Diego (Department of Reproductive Medicine, School of Medicine, University of California San Diego), in Gainesville, Florida (Women's Medical and Diagnostic Center), and Cleveland, Ohio (University MacDonald Women's Hospital). We can only hope that newer clinics all over the country will learn from them.

medical profession and among nonmedical researchers. What you get is one doctor's (or a few doctors') opinions about menopause, based on the women they see and the research they do. Because most doctors are faithful to a medical model of menopause (the model that views it as a "deficiency condition"), and because they rarely see healthy menopausal women, what they have to say may or may not correspond with your own experience. Some women discover that specialists (gynecologists) view menopause so differently that they are better off consulting their family doctors. These sessions often bolster the image of gynecologist as all-knowing, and there is rarely opportunity for discussion of the very real concerns that most women harbor.

These kinds of sessions are popular with women who are reluctant to commit themselves to more than one day or one evening for learning about menopause. The problem is that they may leave more confused than ever. A better bet for those who may not wish to air their problems during the question-and-answer period, and who do not want to listen to the problems of others, is the menopause workshop.

Menopause Workshops

The menopause workshop may also be called a discussion group or seminar, or may appear as part of the course offerings of a Continuing Education or Adult Education section of a local school, college, or university. Whatever its name, the workshop is usually scheduled at a particular time and location, to take place for a specified number of sessions in a neutral setting. Someone trained in group work is hired to facilitate the discussion, and "experts" may be invited to some sessions to explain particular aspects of menopause. Depending on the size of the group and the topics to be covered, there may or may not be ample opportunity to air individual concerns.

The atmosphere in this kind of group depends on the continuing presence of a core group, the duration of the sessions, the number of sessions, how the women interact with each other, and the skills of the facilitator in putting people at ease. It is difficult to predict how satisfying the workshop will be for the individual participant, but the increased demand for such workshops across the country is testimony to their success.

(These kinds of workshops should not be confused with the one-shot workshop that is often held in conjunction with an all-day information session on women's health issues. Often, smaller groups "workshop" on particular topics as a follow-up to a more general information session in the morning.)

A good workshop offers both structured information and moral support—both contribute to the sense that one's menopausal experiences are *not* unique, that one *can* cope, and that menopause is but a temporary disruption. If the structure of an ongoing workshop appeals to you, it may be worth your while to contact some appropriate agencies in your community (your church or synagogue, school boards, community college, women's organization, YWCA, etc.). Often a call is enough to get the ball rolling.

Many women who have attended workshops or discussion groups become so involved with the whole process of group learning that they are inspired to become trained facilitators themselves. Many community women's organizations both encourage and enable their members to learn the skills of facilitating groups, either in courses that they develop themselves or through programs at local colleges or universities.

Some women live too far away from the kinds of institutions that are likely to sponsor menopause workshops. Some women like the idea of the moral support, but are not particularly interested in a review of the physiological processes of menopause and are daunted by the thought of a large group or a classroom. Some women would rather attend sessions at a different time of day, and may be interested in the more informal, and often more intimate self-help group (also known as a mutual aid group or support group).

Self-Help Groups

Self-help groups are formed because the people in them are (or will be) experiencing something in common, and because they want to talk together to help themselves and help each other. Self-help groups are not a substitute for professional help (although they are often a valuable adjunct to professional help) and are not dependent on professional expertise. Self-help groups require a willingness to make the group work, and a commitment from each member of the group to attend the first three or four meetings. Anything else can be decided once the group gets underway.

There are various opinions about the optimum size for a self-help group, but the consensus seems to be in the range of six to twelve. The smaller the group, the more reliant you will be on the commitment of the members to the group; at the same time, smaller groups often foster more intimacy more quickly. Some groups adopt an "open-door" policy, encouraging new members to join the group at any time. Others prefer to encourage intimacy and trust by closing the group, either for a specific number of meetings or for the duration. If the decision is made to close the group, it will require a solid commitment of attendance from each member.

If you wish to start a self-help group, you have various options. You can enlist the help of friends or acquaintances to find members. In other words, from the beginning, you can *share* the job of recruiting. If word-of-mouth is inadequate, you might consider advertising—posting a notice on a bulletin board, placing an ad in a community newspaper or a church bulletin. Your doctor or your friends' doctors may be willing to help by mentioning the idea to likely patients. Sometimes self-help groups can be recruited within the context of a larger meeting. Perhaps an existing women's group will agree to show a film on menopause, or a local organization may be willing to sponsor a presentation about menopause. This provides an opportunity to ask women who attend to sign up if they're interested in a self-help group, or to circulate a "sign-in" sheet and then contact each woman by telephone to see if she (and/or a friend) would be interested in joining the group.

The decision about where to hold the meetings is often a difficult one. The first meeting should be held in a "neutral" place—a school, library, community center, church—some place that's convenient and accessible. You may decide to hold subsequent meetings in each other's homes, but this will depend on the size of the group and the living situation of the members. The meeting places should be protected from interruption from telephone calls, unexpected visitors, and other family members.

No matter how you get started, the first meeting is often taken up with organizational questions. Even when *you* have a clear idea of why you wanted to start a group, you will find that others may have different ideas. It helps if you can articulate and obtain agreement about the general purpose of the group (e.g., "to help us to feel more comfortable about and with menopause"), leaving the precise ways to achieve this to be decided by the group. If the word *menopause* gets in the way of forming a group, a more acceptable goal might be "the exploration of changes in midlife" or something general and nonthreatening. Widow-to-widow groups, or groups for divorced women in their forties or fifties may view menopause as part of a more global objective. Whatever the goal, each member will arrive with her own "hidden agenda"—needs that may or may not be fulfilled by this particular group. In other words, although there may be consensus about the general goal of the self-help group, each person's way of achieving this is likely to be different. This is where the group must formulate specific objectives or tasks to be accomplished at each meeting.

Most self-help groups attempt to meet once a week, but you may find that once every two weeks is more convenient for your members. The meeting itself should run for at least two hours; some groups find that three hours are necessary to allow time for everyone. If coffee (decaffeinated) or herbal tea is served, this should be confined to a short period just before or just after the meeting. Some groups like to set up an agenda in advance, with specific topics slotted for a particular evening. They may also wish to limit the life of the group to a definite number of sessions. (Six is usually the minimum, but some groups aim for eight, or decide to just keep it open-ended.) Other groups prefer to see how much can be covered in one meeting and to spend the last few minutes deciding on the topic for the next. This kind of group may endure for as long as the members feel a need for it.

The thousands of letters that I've received over the years since *A Friend Indeed* was founded tell me that there is one group of women who desperately needs this kind of support: younger women who are dealing with an unexpected and very early menopause, either brought on by surgery or occurring naturally. I know of only one women's center that regularly sponsors such groups. If those of you who work in a women's health center could read, as I do, anguished letters from young women who feel isolated and alone, who cannot understand their own physical and psychological reactions, who are desperate to feel sexual desire, then you would understand why this is so important. Women in their forties don't feel this sense of abandonment because they are more likely to know other women going through the same thing. But if you are in your twenties or thirties, as many women are when menopause is forced upon them, it is hard to know where to turn.

One of the greatest benefits of a group is the new sense of intimacy with women who can empathize with your experience. But women in self-help groups can do much more than express feelings to one another. They can choose to take action about behaviors that contribute, directly or indirectly, to each woman's well-being. Groups of midlife women can get together to exercise, taking "power walks" as a group and then sitting down for a meeting afterwards. Or they can hire a fitness instructor and enjoy a Jazzercise or aerobics class together. Some groups might be interested in learning more about nutrition and practicing recipes based on low-fat or non-fat cooking. Groups such as this might be formed as a way of fostering general good health, or as a way of coping when a family member suffers from some form of cardiovascular disease. Women who house or care for dependent parents often need the aid and support of other women; a group formed around this issue may be of enormous help to other women who find themselves suddenly placed in the same situation.

Together, group members can locate and evaluate doctors in the community, even if the need for doctors' services is not imminent. If a member of the group is apprehensive about a visit to the doctor, another member of the group may go along to offer moral support. There are all sorts of possibilities for a self-help group.

Perhaps this is the greatest gift that menopause brings— the opportunity to reach out to others and to find that, in helping each other, we develop resources, strengths, and abilities we never knew we had.

REFERENCES AND RESOURCES

American Self-Help Clearinghouse, St. Clares-Riverside Medical Center, Denville, NJ 07834 (201-625-7101).

Cobb, J.O. "How to start a menopause self-help group," *A Friend Indeed.* Vol. IV, No. 7, 1987.

Cobb, J.O. "Premature menopause," *A Friend Indeed.* Vol. VIII, No. 9, 1992.

Thomson, Sidney. "Sharing the menopause experience," *Healthsharing:* 10–13, Winter 1986.

Glossary

Adenomyosis Condition where tissue from the endometrium becomes embedded in the muscle of the uterus itself.

Adenosis Abnormal development of a gland.

Adhesions Fibrous tissue that may form in any part of the body as a result of surgery, infection, or bleeding. Adhesions may scar organs together and, when removed surgically, may cause new adhesions to grow.

Adrenal glands Flattened body above both kidneys which produces steroid hormones. The adrenals consist of a cortex and medulla. The cortex is responsible for many hormones; the medulla primarily for epinephrine (adrenaline).

Agoraphobia An irrational fear of being away from a known place. A common phobia among women, agoraphobia is diagnosed when panic attacks dictate a restricted area of activity for the phobic person. It can be effectively treated by behavior therapy.

Air hunger The temporary sensation of being starved of oxygen. Lasting only a few moments, this sensation is characteristic of pregnancy and, more rarely, of menopause.

Alopecia Absence or thinning of hair, a menopausal complaint common to women with a family tendency to male-pattern baldness. No recognized treatment exists although estrogen (too much or too little) may have some influence.

Alopecia areata Patchy hair loss, usually reversible, in sharply defined areas, usually involving the scalp.

Amenorrhea Absence of menstruation for more than three cycles, usually caused by fluctuating estrogen levels during breast feeding, heavy exercise, illness, stress, weight change, or other pattern changes. Episodes of amenorrhea are characteristic of the perimenopause.

Amines Organic compounds containing nitrogen.

Angina Spasmodic, choking, or suffocating pain. Term used almost exclusively for chest pain (angina pectoris) usually due to interference with the supply of oxygen to the heart muscle, precipitated by excitement or effort.

Aneurysm A balloonlike swelling in the walls of a damaged artery.

Anorexia nervosa Condition based on fear of gaining weight, leading to extreme weight loss and amenorrhea. Anorexic patients are typically women in their late teens or early twenties. If not corrected, anorexia can lead to osteoporosis, heart disease and, in some cases, to death by self-starvation.

Apnea The cessation of breathing for a few seconds. Cause is unknown. Sleep apnea is believed responsible for some kinds of very loud snoring and may also be responsible for temporary episodes of "air hunger" during menopause.

Areola Area around the nipple of the breast. May be pink to dark brown.

Arrhythmia Any variation from a regular heartbeat, including tachycardia (too rapid) and bradycardia (too slow).

Arteriosclerosis Hardening of the arteries, a condition in which deposits form inside the arteries and affect blood flow from the heart.

Artery/arteriole Blood vessels that carry freshly oxygenated blood from the heart to all cells of the body.

Aspirated Drained of fluids by suction.

Atheroma Deposit of fats (or lipids) in the artery.

Atherosclerosis The formation of atheromas inside the walls of the arteries; part of the condition known as arteriosclerosis.

Atrophic vaginitis See **Dry vagina**.

Aura A strange sensation that precedes the onset of a hot flash, a migraine headache, or an epileptic seizure. Auras may consist of visual disturbances, feelings of nausea, or sudden changes in mood. The person having the aura learns that it is a signal of the onset of a hot flash, headache, or other atypical sensations.

Basal skin cancer Small, pink growths in the head or neck area. Over time, these change to a cluster of pimples and then to a deep, crusty sore.

Blepharoplasty Medical term for eyelift.

Bloat The sudden distension of the waist or abdomen. Bloat may occur simultaneously with gas, or for no discernible reason. After a period of some discomfort (often two to three hours) it goes away. Common during premenstrual phase and menopause.

Breakthrough bleeding Bleeding or spotting between periods or after a long absence of periods (5 months or more). Should be reported to a doctor.

BSE (Breast self-examination) Practice demonstrated to help identify and minimize effects of breast cancer. BSE done properly once a month can help locate lumps too small to be felt even by an experienced physician.

Bursitis Inflammation of a fluid-filled sac or saclike cavity (bursa). Bursae are situated in places like joints where friction would otherwise occur.

Calcitonin A hormone produced by the thyroid which influences levels of calcium in the blood.

Carcinoma in situ A tumor, the cells of which have not invaded the deepest membrane and are confined to the surface of the organ involved.

Cerebral infarction Death of brain tissue, often as the result of a stroke.

Cerebral thrombosis Blood clot in the brain.

Cerebrovascular accident See **Stroke**.

Cervicitis Inflammation of the neck of the uterus.

Cervix The bottom third of the uterus that projects into the vagina. Viewed through the vagina, the cervix resembles a doughnut.

Cherry angioma Round, bright red spots on the skin made up of blood vessels, often appearing for the first time during middle age.

Cholesterol A substance found in animal fats and oils, egg yolk, and the human body, where it is manufactured by the liver and circulated in the blood.

CHT (Combined Hormone Therapy) Usually understood to comprise ET, or Estrogen Therapy, with the addition of a progestational agent (progestin or progestogen) taken for at least ten days of each cycle *with* the estrogen. Newer regimens comprise daily administration of progestins with estrogen, a course of progestins every three months, or natural progesterones used in suppositories or tablets. CHT is prescribed to women with an intact uterus to protect against endometrial cancer, but is believed to induce more severe side effects than estrogen administered alone. CHT is also known as HRT or Hormone Replacement Therapy.

Climacteric Generally used to refer to the middle years in both males and females, loosely the years from about forty to sixty. The word comes from a Greek term for ladder and signifies a new step every seven years. The climacteric was traditionally the years from forty-two to sixty-three, with the grand climacteric at sixty-three.

Clitoris Female organ of sexual arousal equivalent to male penis.

Clomiphene citrate Generic drug widely known as the fertility drug and prescribed as Clomid, an ovulatory agent that stimulates the release of gonadotropins (FSH and LH).

Clonidine Generic drug prescribed as Catapres, primarily for controlling hypertension but also successful in alleviating hot flashes for 30 percent of the women who try it.

Collagen A main supportive protein of skin, tendon, bone, cartilage, and connective tissue.

Colporrhapy An operation that tightens the supports under the neck of the bladder and removes the slack tissue of the vagina.

Comedomastitis See **Duct ectasia.**

Conization The removal of a cone of tissue from the cervix for inspection and analysis.

Corticosteroid Any of the steroids produced by the adrenal cortex, or other natural or synthetic compounds with similar activity.

Cystitis Inflammation of the bladder, often producing a burning sensation when urinating.

Danazol (Winthrop) The generic term for the drug danocrine, often prescribed for endometriosis, sometimes for PMS. It impedes ovulation and causes a pseudomenopause.

Delestrogen Estrogen used to treat the cessation of menstruation, irregular cycles, abnormal bleeding, menopausal symptoms, and to cause the endometrium to slough off.

Dermabrasion Planing of the skin done by mechanical means (e.g., sandpaper or wire brushes).

Diaphanography Illuminating the breast with a very bright light to reveal the darker masses (potential tumors).

Diastole Force of the heart at rest.

Digitalis A genus of herbs (from the foxglove) used in the treatment of congestive heart failure.

Dry vagina A condition resulting from the thinning out of the vagina walls and occurring either postmenopausally or as a result of surgical menopause (oophorectomy). Also known as *mature vagina*. Unacceptable terms are *atrophic* or *senile vaginitis*.

Duct ectasia Dilation of the collecting (milk) ducts of the breasts. Serious forms of this condition are *comedomastitis* and *plasma cell mastitis*.

Duct hyperplasia Abnormal growth of cells in the lining of the milk ducts of the breasts.

Ductal papillomas Benign growths (warts) in the milk ducts of the breasts.

Emphysema A pathological accumulation of air in tissues or organs.

Endocrine Bodily system comprising glands that release hormones into the bloodstream—that is, pituitary, thyroid, parathryoid, adrenals, pineal body, gonads (ovaries or testes), pancreas, and paraganglia.

Endocrinologist A doctor of internal medicine who specializes in diagnosis and treatment of endocrine gland disorders.

Endometriosis Abnormal occurrence of tissues, which more or less perfectly resemble the endometrium, in various locations in the pelvic cavity.

Endometrium Tissue lining the uterus or womb.

Epidemiologist One who studies the relationships of various factors determining the frequency and distribution of diseases in the human community.

Epidermis The outermost, nonvascular layer of skin.

Ergotamine Tartrate salt used for the relief of migraine.

ERT (Estrogen Replacement Therapy) See **ET (Estrogen Therapy)**.

Estrace (Mead Johnson) Estrogen used in ET, given cyclically, often coupled with progestogen/androgen to prevent buildup of endometrial tissue. Prescribed for the relief of menopausal symptoms.

Estraderm (Ciba-Geigy) Patch containing a reservoir of estrogen that seeps through the skin into the bloodstream, avoiding metabolism by the liver.

Estradiol　A strong estrogen produced by the ovaries. The major estrogen in premenopausal women.

Estriol　The least powerful form of estrogen, a byproduct of estrone.

Estrogen　Hormone classified as "female sex hormone" although it is produced by both men and women. There are three different kinds of hormones, the major one, estradiol, is produced in the ovaries.

Estrone　A weak hormone produced partly by the ovaries and partly through the conversion, in body fat, of a precursor from the adrenal glands. Estrone is the main postmenopausal estrogen, and the conversion process becomes more efficient with age.

ET (Estrogen Therapy)　The most common form of supplementary estrogen prescribed, usually consisting of one tablet (to be taken orally) once a day for 25 days, with the balance of the month off. Continuous (noncyclical) ET is an alternative regimen. ET is also available via patches (see **Estraderm**) and, where approved, pellets, gels, and vaginal rings. The common term, Estrogen Replacement Therapy (ERT), is only appropriate where endogenous estrogen is no longer available as the result of surgery, radiation, or chemotherapy, and exogenous estrogens are required. See also **CHT**.

Ethinyl estradiol　A common form of synthetic estrogen used in the contraceptive pill and, in much smaller quantities, in some forms of ET.

Fallopian tubes　Tubes with hairlike ends that pick up eggs erupting from the ovary and carry them down into the uterus.

Fibrocystic　Characterized by an overgrowth of fibrous tissue and development of cystic spaces, especially in a gland.

Fibroids　Colloquial clinical term for leiomyoma (benign tumors most often derived from smooth muscle) in or around the uterus.

Fibromyalgia　A "sore-all-over" condition, also referred to as *fibrositis*. Symptoms include aching, pain, stiffness, and sore spots that may continue for months or years. Treated with antiinflammatory drugs, exercise, and relaxation.

Fibrosis   Firm mass in the breasts, difficult to distinguish from normal tissue, usually benign.

Fibrous dysplasia   See **Fibrosis.**

Follicle   Seed pod, or pouchlike covering surrounding the egg, or ovum, produced by the ovaries. When the follicle bursts, an egg is released to be picked up by the fallopian tubes.

Formication   A word used to describe the sensation of ants crawling on the skin, a common experience during menopause.

Geriatrics   Branch of medicine dealing with the problems of aging and diseases of the elderly.

Gerontology   The scientific study of the problems of aging in all its aspects.

Giant fibroadenoma   Rapidly growing rubbery tumor in the breast.

Gonadotropin   A substance that has a stimulating effect upon the ovaries, especially the hormone secreted by the anterior pituitary. Comprises Follicle Stimulating Hormone (FSH) and Luteinizing Hormone (LH).

Histamine   Amine that causes dilation of capillaries, constriction of the muscles in the lungs, and increased gastric secretion.

Hormone   Substance produced by a gland and circulating through the bloodstream.

Hot flash   The subjective sensation of heat, often through the chest and over the head but felt, by some women, to the ends of their fingertips and to the soles of the feet. There may be an accompanying rise in temperature. The most common menopausal complaint in Western societies, the cause of the hot flash is unknown. (In Britain, "flush" is used in place of "flash.")

Hot flush   The evidence (red neck, face, enlarged veins, etc.)

that often accompanies a hot flash. Not all hot flashes produce a flush. Not all flushes are felt as a flash.

HRT (Hormone Replacement Therapy) See **CHT (Combined Hormone Therapy)**.

Hyperplasia Abnormal increase in the number of normal cells in normal arrangement in an organ or tissue, which increases in volume.

Hysterectomy Surgical removal of the uterus. A complete hysterectomy involves removal of the uterus and cervix. A partial hysterectomy involves removal of the uterus only. A radical hysterectomy involves removal of uterus, cervix, lymph nodes, and sometimes part of the vagina.

Hysteroscope A fiber optic instrument used to examine the cervical canal and uterine cavity.

Introductal papillomas Wartlike growths in the breast that may produce a discharge from the nipple.

Labia Lips (outer and inner) that cover female genitals.

Laparoscopy Procedure that may be diagnostic or operative. When used for diagnosis, it involves examination of the abdominal or pelvic cavity. A small incision is made in the navel, and carbon dioxide or nitrous oxide is pumped into the abdomen to give the doctor a better view of the pelvic organs. A laparoscope is then inserted, through which the doctor examines the pelvic organs. A second incision on the pubic line may be required for operative laparoscopy.

Laparotomy Incision through the abdominal wall.

Lipectomy Medical term for fat suction (lipolysis).

Lipoma A benign fatty tumor usually composed of mature fat cells.

Lipoprotein A combination of a lipid and a protein, having the general properties of proteins, but categorized as high density, low density, or very low density (HDLs, LDLs, VLDLs).

Lithotomy Incision of a duct or organ for the removal of abnormal growths.

Lithotomy position Term used to describe the position of a woman during standard gynecological examination (i.e., knees spread, feet up on stirrups). This position is also used for certain types of hysterectomies, particularly for prolapsed uterus, but may also involve tipping of the operating table so that the surgeon has a better view of the operating field. This often results in severe postoperative backache for the patient.

Lorazepam Generic tranquilizer prescribed for relief of excessive anxiety. Often prescribed to menopausal women, lorazepam is addictive and acts as a depressant.

Lypolysis Medical term for fat suction.

Malignant melanoma Form of cancer resulting from overexposure to the sun. It begins as a raised, bumpy, darkened area of skin. Its shape and color may change, and it may be itchy or sore.

Mastitis Inflammation of the breast.

Menopause Medical definition: the cessation of menstruation. Nonmedical definition: the years surrounding the cessation of menstruation.

Menrium Esterified estrogen and diazepam (tranquilizer) sometimes prescribed for menopausal women. Addictive.

Mitral valve The valve between the left atrium and the left ventricle of the heart.

Naturopathy A drugless system of healing by the use of physical methods.

Necrosis Hard lump consisting of dead cells, often resulting from a blow.

Oophorectomy Excision of one or both ovaries.

Osteoarthritis Degenerative joint disease accompanied by pain and stiffness.

Osteomalacia Softening of the bones due to a vitamin D deficiency.

Osteopenia Any condition involving reduced bone mass.

Osteoporosis Abnormal rarefaction of bone; porous bones.

Palpitations Disagreeable subjective awareness of the heart beating.

Perimenopause Period of time surrounding menopause when menstruation is irregular.

Petrolatum A purified mixture of hydrocarbons obtained from petroleum used as an ointment base or soothing application to the skin.

Phlebitis Inflammation of a vein.

Placebo Inactive substance given to satisfy a need for drug therapy, or to compare effects in one group with effects of an active substance given to another group.

Plasma cell mastitis See **Duct ectasia.**

Postmenopause Period of time when menstruation has definitely ceased. Postmenopause is usually understood to begin when a woman has not had a menstrual period for twelve months.

Premarin (Ayerst) Conjugated estrogen in oral tablets, used in ET. Often prescribed in conjunction with synthetic progesterone (Provera).

Premenopause Period of time when signs of menopause are present but before menstrual periods become irregular.

Premenstrual syndrome (PMS) A wide range of physical and emotional symptoms that precede (by usually seven to ten days) the menstrual period.

Prodrome See **Aura.**

Progesterone Hormone produced by the corpus luteum (yellow body) which is left after a follicle bursts from the ovary. This hormone paves the way for menstruation.

Progestin Synthetic form of progesterone. Generic names are medroxyprogesterone acetate and megestrol acetate.

Progestogen Synthetic hormone derived from the male hormone, testosterone. Generic names are norethindrone or norethisterone.

Prostate A gland surrounding the neck of the bladder and urethra in the male; it contributes a secretion to the semen.

Provera (Upjohn) Trademark name of progestogens that cause the endometrium to shed. May be prescribed to accompany estrogen (to control severe menopausal symptoms) or to help regulate unusual bleeding.

Reserpine   An alkaloid used as an antihypertensive and tranquilizer.

Rhytidectomy   Medical term for a facelift.

Rickets   A condition caused by vitamin D deficiency. Bones do not harden normally but are bent and distorted, and the bones have enlarged nodes at the ends and sides.

Senile lentigos   Liver spots caused by melanin (the dark pigment of the skin) deposits.

Sonography   See **Ultrasound**.

Spironolactone   An aldosterone (steroid hormone) inhibitor primarily prescribed as a diuretic.

Squamous cell cancer   Form of cancer that starts as a small, red, hard pimple and then becomes a hard, crusted sore that refuses to heal.

Stilbestrol   Synthetic nonsteroidal estrogen. Effects are similar to those of natural estrogens. Once used to prevent miscarriage, to dry up breast milk, and as a morning-after pill. Its legal use is now limited to the treatment of breast and prostate cancer.

Stroke   A condition with sudden onset due to acute vascular lesions of the brain (hemorrhage, embolism, thrombosis, rupturing aneurysm), which may be marked by partial or total paralysis of one side of the body, vertigo, numbness, or partial or total loss of speech, often followed by permanent neurologic damage. Medical terms are CVA (cerebrovascular accident) or, in its milder form, TIA (transient ischemic accident).

Suction currettage   Another term for fat suction.

Systole   Force of the heart while pumping.

Temporomandibular jaw syndrome (TMJ)   Faulty articulation of the hinged joint of the jaw; a condition that may cause, in addition to headache, dizziness or ringing in the ears.

Testosterone   A hormone secreted primarily in the male testes, which functions in the induction and maintenance of male secondary sex characteristics. Also produced in minute quantities in the female ovaries. Synthetic testosterone is made from cholesterol or isolated from bull testes.

Thermography Diagnostic technique that measures temperature differences between normal and abnormal (warmer) tissues. Useful but, by itself, not accurate enough for diagnosing breast cancer.

Thromboembolism Obstruction of a blood vessel with thrombotic material carried by the blood from the site of origin to plug another vessel.

Touch impairment Sensitivity to being touched which makes one shrink from human contact or impedes responses to touch. Usually temporary. Treatable with ET.

Transillumination See **Diaphanography.**

Tubal ligation Surgical technique of sterilization. The fallopian tubes are cut and bound, or plugged. Rarely reversible.

Ultrasound Technique that sends sound waves into the body that are reflected back onto a screen for display.

Uterus A muscular organ, pear-sized and shaped, part of the same structure as the cervix. Also known as the womb. The lining of the uterus is the endometrium. As well as holding the developing fetus, the uterus produces a substance called prostacyclin, which may influence the capacity for sexual response.

Vasodilator Any agent which causes dilation of blood vessels.

Vitamin E Fat soluble vitamin stored in the liver, fatty tissues, heart, muscles, testes, uterus, blood, and adrenal and pituitary glands.

Withdrawal bleed An artificial menstrual period, induced by CHT, assumed to eliminate the buildup of excess cells in the uterus.

Bibliography

Each chapter in this book is followed by a list of references and resources which are pertinent to the material covered in that chapter. Following are books, articles and other resources which are helpful in extending general knowledge about menopause.

Anderson, M. *The Menopause*, London: Faber and Faber, 1983.

Anderson, E., S. Hamburger, J. Lui, and R. Rebar. "Characteristics of menopausal women seeking assistance," *Am. J. Obs. Gynecol.*, 156(2):438–443, 1987.

Ballinger, S. E. and W. L. Walker. *Not the Change of Life: Breaking the menopause taboo.* Ringwood, Australia: Penguin, 1987.

Bart, P. B. and M. Grossman. "Menopause," *Women & Health*, 1(2):3–10, 1976.

Baruch, G. and J. Brooks-Gunn, eds. *Women in Midlife.* NY: Plenum Press, 1984.

Beard, M. and L. Curtis. *Menopause and the Years Ahead.* Tucson: Fisher, 1988.

Berger, H. and M. Boulet, eds. *A Portrait of the Menopause: Expert reports on medical and therapeutic strategies for the 1990s.* Park Ridge, NJ: Parthenon, 1991.

Beyene, Y. *From Menarche to Menopause.* Albany, NY: State University of New York Press, 1989.

Borton, J. C. *Drawing from the Women's Well: Reflections on the life passage of menopause.* San Diego, CA: LuraMedia, 1992.

Boston Women's Health Book Collective. *The New Our Bodies Ourselves (rev. ed.).* NY: Simon & Schuster, 1992.

Budoff, P. W. *No More Hot Flashes and Other Good News.* NY: Putnam, 1983.

Burg, D. and M. J. Minkin. *What's Stopped Happening to Me?* NY: Carol Publishing, 1990.

Burnett, R. G. *Menopause: All your questions answered.* Chicago: Contemporary Books, 1987.

Butler, R. and M. Lewis. *Love and Sex After Forty: A guide for men and women in their mid- and later years.* NY: Harper & Row, 1986.

Cherry, S. *The Menopause Myth.* NY: Ballantine, 1976.

Clay, V. S. *Women: Menopause and Middle Age.* Pittsburgh: Know Inc., 1977.

Cohen, J. Z., K. L. Coburn, and J. Pearlman. *Hitting Our Stride: Good news about women in their middle years.* NY: Delacorte Press, 1980.

Coope, J. *The Menopause: Coping with the change.* NY: Prentice-Hall, 1984.

Corea, G. *Women's Health Care: The hidden malpractice.* NY: Morrow, 1977.

Cutler, W. B. and C. R. Garcia. *Menopause: A Guide for women and the men who love them (rev. ed.).* NY: Norton, 1992.

Cutler, W. B. and C. R. Garcia. *The Medical Management of Menopause and Premenopause.* Philadelphia: Lippincott, 1984.

Dawson, D. *Women's Cancers: The treatment options—everything you need to know.* London: Judy Piatkus, 1990.

DeMarco, C. *For Women Only: Take charge of your body (3rd ed.).* Winlaw, B.C.: The Last Laugh, 1990.

Doress, P. B. and D. L. Siegal (and the Midlife and Older Women Book Project). *Ourselves, Growing Older.* NY: Simon & Schuster, 1987.

Downing, C. *Journey through Menopause: A personal rite of passage.* NY: Crossroad Publishing, 1987.

Dranov, P. *Estrogen: Is It Right For You?* NY: Fireside, 1993.

Dreifus, C., ed. *Seizing Our Bodies: The politics of women's health.* NY: Random House, 1977.

Ehrenreich, B. and D. English. *Complaints and Disorders: The sexual politics of sickness* (Glass Mountain Pamphlet No. 2). Brooklyn, NY: Faculty Press, 1973.

Ehrenreich, B. and D. English. *For Her Own Good: 150 years of the experts' advice to women.* NY: Anchor, 1979.

Evans, B. *Life Change: A guide to the menopause, its effects and treatment.* London: Pan Books, 1979.

Fausto-Sterling, A. *Myths of Gender: Biological theories about women and men.* NY: Basic Books, 1985.

Feltin, M. *A Woman's Guide to Good Health After 50.* Glenview, IL: Scott Foresman, 1987.

Ford, G. *What's Wrong With My Hormones?* New Castle, CA: Desmond Ford, 1992.

Formanek, R., ed. *The Meanings of Menopause: Historical, medical and clinical perspectives.* Hillsdale, NJ: Analytic Press, 1990.

A Friend Indeed: For women in the prime of life (monthly newsletter), Box 1710, Champlain, NY 12919–1710.

Frisch, M. *Stay Cool Through Menopause: Answers to your most-asked questions.* Los Angeles: The Body Press, 1989.

Gannon, L. R. *Menstrual Disorders and Menopause: Biological, psychological and cultural research.* NY: Praeger, 1985.

Gillespie, C. *Hormones, Hot Flashes and Mood Swings: Living through the ups and downs of menopause.* NY: Harper & Row, 1989.

Gray, M. *The Changing Years: The Menopause Without Fear.* NY: Doubleday, 1991.

Greenblatt, R. *The Menopausal Syndrome.* NY: Medcom Press, 1974.

Greenwood, S. *Menopause Naturally: Preparing for the second half of your life (3rd ed.).* San Francisco: Volcano Press, 1992.

Greer, G. *The Change: Women, aging and the menopause.* NY: Knopf, 1992.

Grist, L. *A Woman's Guide to Alternative Medicine.* Chicago, IL: Contemporary Books, 1988.

Hailes, J., R. J. Doran and P. A. Lum-Doran. *Middle Years: The Female Menopause.* Toronto: Copp Clark Pitman, 1982.

Henig, R. M. *How A Woman Ages: What to expect and what you can do about it.* NY: Ballantine, 1985.

Hot Flash (quarterly newsletter), National Action Forum for Midlife and Older Women, Box 815, Stony Brook, NY 11790-0609.

Hunter, M. *Your Menopause.* London: Pandora, 1990.

Jacobowitz, R. S. *150 Most-Asked Questions About Menopause.* NY: Hearst, 1993.

Jovanovic, L. and G. J. Subak-Sharpe. *Hormones: The woman's answerbook.* NY: Fawcett Columbine, 1987.

Kahn, A. P. and L. H. Holt. *Midlife Health.* NY: Facts on File, 1987.

Kaufert, P. and J. Syrotiuk. "Symptom reporting at the menopause", *Soc. Sci. Med., 151:*173–184, 1981.

Khatchadourian, H. *Fifty: Midlife in perspective.* NY: Freeman, 1987.

Lark, S. M. *The Menopause Self-Help Book.* Berkeley, CA: Celestial Arts, 1990.

London, S. and H. J. Chihal. *Menopause: Clinical concepts.* NY: Essential Medical Information Systems, 1989.

Lopez, M. C. et al. *Menopause: A self-care manual.* 1989. Santa Fe Health Education Project, P. O. Box 577, Santa Fe, New Mexico 87502.

MacPherson, K. I. "Menopause as disease: The social construction of a metaphor," *Annals of Nursing Sci., 3:*95–113, 1981.

McCrea, F. B. "The politics of menopause: The 'discovery' of a deficiency disease," *Social Problems, 31*(1), 1983.

Mankowitz, A. *Change of Life: A psychological study of dreams and the menopause.* Toronto: Inner City Books, 1984.

Martin, E. *The Woman in the Body: A cultural analysis of reproduction.* Boston: Beacon Press, 1987.

Mastroianni, L., Jr. and C. A. Paulsen, eds. *Aging, Reproduction and the Climacteric.* NY: Plenum Press, 1986.

Maturitas: International journal for the study of the climacteric. Elsevier Science Publishers, Box 211, 1000 AE Amsterdam, The Netherlands.

Melpomene Report, Melpomene Institute for Women's Health Research, 1010 University Avenue, St. Paul, MN 55104.

Melville, A. *Natural Hormone Health: Drug-free ways to manage your life.* London: Thorsons, 1990.

Menopause News (bi-monthly newsletter), 2074 Union St., San Francisco, CA 94123.

Midlife Woman (bi-monthly newsletter), Midlife Women's Network, 5129 Logan Ave. South, Minneapolis, MN 55419-1019.

Millette, B. and J. Hawkins. *The Passage Through Menopause: Women's Lives in Transition.* VA: Reston Publishing, 1983.

Montreal Health Press. *Menopause: A well woman book.* Toronto: Second Story Press, 1990.

Musgrave, B. and Z. Menell, eds. *Change and Choice: Women and middle age.* London: Peter Owen, 1980.

Nachtigall, L. and J. R. Heilman. *Estrogen: The facts can change your life.* Tucson: The Body Press, 1986.

Nellis, M. *The Female Fix.* NY: Penguin Books, 1980.

The Network News (quarterly newsletter), The National Women's Health Network, 1325 G St. N.W., Lower Level, Washington, D.C. 20005.

Neugarten, B. *Middle Age and Aging.* Chicago: University of Chicago Press, 1968.

Ojeda, L. *Menopause without Medicine.* Claremont, CA: Hunter House, 1989.

Paige, J. and P. Gordon. *Choice Years.* NY: Villard, 1991.

Perry, S. and K. O'Hanlan. *Natural Menopause.* NY: Addison-Wesley, 1992.

Porcino, J. *Growing Older, Getting Better.* NY: Addison-Wesley, 1983.

Porcino, J. *Living Longer, Living Better: Adventures in community housing for those in the second half of life.* NY: Continuum, 1991.

Reimer, B. L. *The Menopausal Years.* Daly City, CA: Krames Communications, 1980.

Rose, L., ed. *The Menopause Book.* NY: Hawthorn, 1977.

Sachs, J. *What Women Should Know About Menopause.* NY: Dell, 1991.

Schoenfeld, O. and B. B. Smith. *Change for the Better: Preparing for the Freedom of Menopause.* Old Tappan, NJ: Fleming H. Revell, 1979.

Schwartz, D. P., ed. *Hormone Replacement Therapy.* Baltimore: Williams & Wilkins, 1992.

Scully, D. H. *Men Who Control Women's Health.* Boston: Houghton, Mifflin, 1980.

Sheehy, G. *The Silent Passage: Menopause.* NY: Random House, 1991.

Shreeve, C. M. *Overcoming the Menopause Naturally.* London: Arrow Books, 1986.

Sitruk-Ware, R. and W. Utian, eds. *The Menopause and Hormone Replacement Therapy: Facts and controversies.* NY: Marcel Dekker, 1991.

Smith, J. *Women and Doctors.* NY: Atlantic Monthly Press, 1992.

SMCR Newsletter (quarterly newsletter), Society for Menstrual Cycle Research, c/o Mary Anna Friederich, M.D., 10559 N. 104th Place, Scottsdale, AZ 85258.

Taylor, D. and A. C. Sumrall. *Women of the 14th Moon.* Freedom, CA: Crossing Press, 1991.

Trien, S. F. *The Menopause Handbook.* NY: Fawcett, Columbine, 1986. (Originally issued as *Change of Life.*)

U.S. Congress, Office of Technology Assessment. *Menopause, Hormone Therapy & Women's Health,* OTA-BP-BA-88, Washington DC: US Government Printing Office, 1992.

U.S. Congress, Select Committee on Aging. *Staying Healthy, Being Aware: Health Care After Forty,* ISBN 0–16–038404–4. Washington, DC: U.S. Government Printing Office, 1992.

Ussher, J. M. *Psychology of the Female Body.* NY: Routledge, 1989.

Utian, W. and R. S. Jacobowitz. *Managing Your Menopause.* Englewood Cliffs, NJ: Prentice Hall, 1990.

Voda, A. M., M. Dinnerstein, and S. R. O'Donnell, eds. *Changing Perspectives on Menopause.* Austin: University of Texas Press, 1982.

Weideger, P. *Menstruation & Menopause: The physiology and psychology, the myth and the reality.* NY: Knopf, 1976.

Weiss, K., ed. *Women's Health Care: A guide to alternatives.* Reston, VA: Reston, 1984.

Wells, R. G. and M. C. Wells. *Menopause and Mid-Life.* Wheaton, IL: Tyndale House, 1990.

Wilson, R. A. *Feminine Forever.* NY: Pocket Books, 1968.

Wolfe, S. M. *Women's Health Alert.* NY: Addison-Wesley, 1991.

Women's Health Journal (English or Spanish), Isis International: the Latin American and Caribbean Women's Health Network, Casilla 2067, Correo Centrale, Santiago, Chile.

Zichella, L., M. I. Whitehead, and P. A. Van Keep, eds. *The Climacteric and Beyond.* Park Ridge, NJ: Parthenon, 1988.

Index

Codeine, 54
Cod liver oil. *See* Vitamin D
Coffee:
  caffeine in. *See* Caffeine
  methylxamine in, 147
Colas:
  caffeine in. *See* Caffeine
  methylxamine in, 147
Collagen, 253–54
Collagen injections, 49, 253
Colon cancer, 204
Colporrhapy, 173
Colposcopy, 174–75
Combined hormone therapy (CHT),
    9*n.*, 84, 92, 155
  contraindications, 99–100
  deciding on, 107–11
  heart disease and, 105
  history of, 91–92
  for hot flashes, 100, 108
  methods of prescribing, 92–98
    charts, 94–97
  monthly bleed, 98
  noncompliance, 106
  popularity of, 92
  reasons for prescribing, 100–05
  regular medical examinations
    and, 108
  side effects, 97, 106–07
Comedomastitis, 149
Cone biopsy, 174
Congestive heart failure, 200
Congressional Subcommittee
    Hearing on menopause, xiii
Constipation, 42, 76, 204, 207
Coronary heart disease (CHD), 134
Coronary thrombosis, 132
Corpus luteum, 88
Cortical bone, 117
Corticosteroids, 32, 114
Cortisone, 26
Cortisone cream, 50
Cosmetics, 258, 264
Cosmetic surgeons, 253
  questions to ask, 261
  selecting, 261
Cosmetic surgery, 259–63
  body contouring, 259

contraindications, 259
  on the eyes, 263
  facelifts, 259, 262–63
  fat suction, 259–61
  negative outcomes, 261
  See also Cosmetic surgeons
Counselors, 33, 75
Cramps:
  hormone therapy and, 106
  menstrual, 40
  muscle, 117–22
Crying, unexplained, 20
Cryosurgery, 174
Cultural definitions of menopause,
    12–14
Cushing's syndrome, 114
Cystic hyperplasia, 176
Cystitis, 20, 24, 44
  medication for, 50, 102
  nonprescription remedies, 48–49
Cystosarcoma phyllodes, 148
Cysts, breast. *See* Breasts, cysts

Dairy products, 47
  calcium absorption and, 125
  milk, 206
  yogurt, 47, 48, 56, 57
Danazol (danocrine), 166, 169
D&C. *See* dilatation and curettage
Decaffeinated beverages, 199
Densitometry, 123
Dental cavities, 200
Dental work, 136–37, 258
Depilatory, 257
Depression, 2, 9, 11, 14, 19, 20,
    71–76
  bipolar (manic), 72
  clonidine and, 42
  exercise and, 74, 197, 207
  after hysterectomy, 9, 72, 185
  methods of fighting, 74–76,
    100–01
  night sweats and, 23
  postpartum, 74
  as self-limiting, 72, 76
Dermabrasion, 263
Dermatologists, 251, 253
DES, 90, 91, 158–59, 204